Musculoskeletal Examination of the Foot and Ankle

Making the Complex Simple

Edited by

Shepard R. Hurwitz, MD
Professor of Orthopaedic Surgery
Department of Orthopaedics
University of North Carolina Health System
Chapel Hill, North Carolina

Selene G. Parekh, MD, MBA
Associate Professor of Orthopaedic Surgery
Department of Orthopaedic Surgery
Duke University
North Carolina Orthopaedic Clinic
Adjunct Faculty
Fuqua Business School
Durham, North Carolina

Musculoskeletal Examination
Making the Complex Simple
Series

Series Editor, Steven B. Cohen, MD

SLACK
INCORPORATED

www.slackbooks.com

ISBN: 978-1-55642-919-4

The procedures and practices described in this publication should be implemented in a manner consistent with the professional standards set for the circumstances that apply in each specific situation. Every effort has been made to confirm the accuracy of the information presented and to correctly relate generally accepted practices. The authors, editors, and publisher cannot accept responsibility for errors or exclusions or for the outcome of the material presented herein. There is no expressed or implied warranty of this book or information imparted by it. Care has been taken to ensure that drug selection and dosages are in accordance with currently accepted/recommended practice. Off-label uses of drugs may be discussed. Due to continuing research, changes in government policy and regulations, and various effects of drug reactions and interactions, it is recommended that the reader carefully review all materials and literature provided for each drug, especially those that are new or not frequently used. Some drugs or devices in this publication have clearance for use in a restricted research setting by the Food and Drug and Administration or FDA. Each professional should determine the FDA status of any drug or device prior to use in their practice.

Any review or mention of specific companies or products is not intended as an endorsement by the author or publisher.

SLACK Incorporated uses a review process to evaluate submitted material. Prior to publication, educators or clinicians provide important feedback on the content that we publish. We welcome feedback on this work.

Published by: SLACK Incorporated
6900 Grove Road
Thorofare, NJ 08086 USA
Telephone: 856-848-1000
Fax: 856-848-6091
www.slackbooks.com

Contact SLACK Incorporated for more information about other books in this field or about the availability of our books from distributors outside the United States.

Library of Congress Cataloging-in-Publication Data

Musculoskeletal examination of the foot and ankle : making the complex simple / edited by Shepard R. Hurwitz, Selene G. Parekh.
p. ; cm. -- (Musculoskeletal examination : making the complex simple series)
Includes bibliographical references and index.
ISBN 978-1-55642-919-4 (pbk.)
1. Foot--Diseases--Diagnosis. 2. Ankle--Diseases--Diagnosis. 3. Musculoskeletal system--Diseases--Diagnosis. I. Hurwitz, Shepard R. II. Parekh, Selene G. III. Series: Musculoskeletal examination : making the complex simple series.
[DNLM: 1. Foot Diseases--diagnosis. 2. Ankle--pathology. 3. Diagnostic Techniques and Procedures. 4. Musculoskeletal Diseases--diagnosis. WE 880]
RC563.M88 2012
616.5'79--dc23

2011026532

Printed in the United States of America.

Last digit is print number: 10 9 8 7 6 5 4 3 2 1

Dedication

For Zoe, who moves and dances with a magic spirit.
For Leah, who is the world explorer we wish we could be.
For Mom, who taught me how to communicate in writing.

Shepard R. Hurwitz, MD

To my parents, Gunvant and Bharati Parekh, who instilled traditional values; emphasized the importance of family, hard work, and education; and created opportunities for me.

To my brother, Jai, who provides wisdom and guidance.

To my wife, Zankhna, who provides me with support, encouragement, and advice and is my beacon in life.

To my children, Aarav, Arsh, and Anaya, for the inspiration, happiness, enthusiasm, and joy they bring.

Selene G. Parekh, MD, MBA

Contents

Acknowledgments

To Dr. N. Lynn Gerber, my sister, who has devoted a career toward improving the lives of many who were impaired or disabled, and whose knowledge of the foot and ankle rivals that of any orthopedist.

To J. Leonard Goldner, who taught in many ways what to do, how to do, and when to do, and to always do your best for the patient.

Shepard R. Hurwitz, MD

I would like to acknowledge my mentor and friend, Keith L. Wapner, MD. He ignited the passion of foot and ankle surgery in me and reinforced the importance of family above all else.

Selene G. Parekh, MD, MBA

About the Editors

Shepard R. Hurwitz, MD is a professor of orthopedic surgery in the Department of Orthopaedics at the University of North Carolina Health System, Chapel Hill, North Carolina. Dr. Hurwitz has been involved with medical student and resident education, basic and clinical research, patient care, and medical center administration for nearly 30 years. He has practiced orthopedic foot and ankle surgery since completing a year of postdoctoral fellowship, in private practice, in government service (US Army and Veterans Administration) and in 4 different residency teaching programs. He has several teaching and service awards from the American Academy of Orthopaedic Surgeons, the American Diabetes Association, the Orthopaedic Research and Education Foundation, the University of Virginia, George Washington University, and National Institutes of Health. Author or coauthor of more than 80 manuscripts, 14 book chapters, and editor of 4 texts on foot and ankle surgery, his main area of clinical interest is in outcomes following surgery of the ankle and hindfoot.

Selene G. Parekh, MD, MBA is an associate professor of orthopedic surgery at the North Carolina Orthopaedic Clinic and Duke University, Department of Orthopaedic Surgery. His research and clinical interests include total ankle replacements, foot and ankle injuries of athletes, minimally invasive foot and ankle trauma surgery, tendon injuries of the foot and ankle, and the adoption and development of novel technologies in foot and ankle surgery. He has been an active speaker at regional, national, and international meetings, helping to teach other orthopedic surgeons about novel techniques for the care of foot and ankle patients.

Contributing Authors

Ian Alexander, MD, FRCS(C) (Chapter 1)
Professor, Department of Orthopaedic Surgery
Ohio State University
Columbus, Ohio

Wayne Berberian, MD (Chapter 10)
Associate Professor of Orthopedics
UMDNJ New Jersey Medical School
Department of Orthopedics
Newark, New Jersey

Eric Breitbart, MD (Chapter 10)
Orthopedic Resident
UMDNJ New Jersey Medical School
Department of Orthopedics
Newark, New Jersey

Christopher P. Chiodo, MD (Chapter 8)
Foot and Ankle Division Chief
Department of Orthopedic Surgery
Brigham and Women's Hospital
Harvard Medical School
Boston, Massachusetts

Premjit S. Deol, DO (Chapter 11)
Panorama Orthopedics and Spine Center
Golden, Colorado

Antonio Gomez-Tristan, MD (Chapter 8)
Foot and Ankle Fellow
Harvard Medical School
Department of Orthopaedics
Brigham and Women´s Hospital
Boston, Massachusetts

Adam T. Groth, MD (Chapter 7)
MAJ, MC, USA
Orthopaedic Surgery Service
Tripler Army Medical Center
Honolulu, Hawaii

Sheldon Lin, MD (Chapter 10)
Associate Professor of Orthopedics
UMDNJ- New Jersey Medical School
Department of Orthopedics
Newark, New Jersey

James Meeker, MD (Chapter 5)
Chief Resident
Orthopaedic Surgery
University of North Carolina
Chapel Hill, North Carolina

Samir Mehta, MD (Chapter 9)
Chief, Orthopaedic Trauma & Fracture Services
Hospital of the University of Pennsylvania
Assistant Professor, Department of Orthopaedic Surgery
University of Pennsylvania School of Medicine
Philadelphia, Pennsylvania

David I. Pedowitz, MD (Chapter 3)
Department of Orthopedic Surgery
Crystal Run Healthcare
Middletown, New York

Terrence M. Philbin, DO (Chapter 11)
Attending Physician
Orthopedic Foot and Ankle Center
Westerville, Ohio
Director, Foot and Ankle Service
Doctors Hospital Residency
Columbus, Ohio

Seth R. Queler, MD (Chapter 4)
Attending Physician
Orthopaedic Surgeon
Femino-Ducey Orthopaedic Group
Clara Maass Medical Center
Department of Orthopaedic Surgery
Belleville, New Jersey

Sudheer Reddy, MD (Chapter 2)
Orthopedic Surgeon
Frederick Memorial Hospital
Frederick, Maryland

Lew Schon, MD (Chapter 7)
Chief Foot & Ankle Fellowship and Orthobiologic Laboratory
Union Memorial Hospital
Baltimore, Maryland
Orthopaedic and Dance Science Consultant
Goucher College
Towson, Maryland
Assistant Professor Orthopaedics
Johns Hopkins School of Medicine
Baltimore, Maryland
Assistant Professor Biomedical Engineering
Johns Hopkins University
Baltimore, Maryland
Associate Professor of Orthopaedics
Georgetown School of Medicine
Washington, DC
President Elect
American Orthopaedic Foot and Ankle Society

Aaron T. Scott, MD (Chapter 12)
Assistant Professor
Department of Orthopaedic Surgery
Wake Forest University School of Medicine
Winston-Salem, North Carolina

Joshua N. Tennant, MD, MPH (Chapter 5)
Department of Orthopaedic Surgery (PGY-5)
University of North Carolina Hospitals
Chapel Hill, North Carolina

Keith Wapner, MD (Chapter 6)
Clinical Professor, Orthopedic Surgery
University of Pennsylvania
Adjunct Professor, Orthopedic Surgery
Drexel College of Medicine
Director, Foot and Ankle Fellowship Program
University of Pennsylvania
Philadelphia, Pennsylvania

Foreword

The foot and ankle are made up of 26 bones and 33 joints powered and stabilized by over 100 muscles, tendons, and ligaments. This intricate machinery serves as a foundation for shock absorption, accommodation, and ambulation. Despite the small surface areas, the foot and ankle articulations receive the largest forces in the body allowing us to walk, run, and jump. Understanding this complex musculoskeletal unit can be overwhelming to students and medical providers.

Drs. Shepard R. Hurwitz and Selene G. Parekh are to be commended for writing *Musculoskeletal Examination of the Foot and Ankle: Making the Complex Simple*. They have compiled chapters from expert orthopedic foot and ankle surgeons who make the complex simple through a standard organized format that is easy to follow, concise, and well written. Readers are walked along descriptions of the foot and ankle physical exam, imaging, and common conditions using supplemental figures and clinical pictures to enhance a point.

With the current boom of information technology and the intricacies of foot and ankle, students and medical practitioners are inundated with details. *Musculoskeletal Examination of the Foot and Ankle: Making the Complex Simple* is an essential resource for the clinicians and an easy, readable tool for the students. Congratulations Drs. Hurwitz and Parekh!

Judith F. Baumhauer, MD, MPH
Professor and Associate Chair of Academic Affairs
Department of Orthopaedic Surgery
Foot and Ankle Division
University of Rochester School of Medicine and Dentistry
Rochester, New York

Introduction

This book is the product of a conversation with Dr. Steven B. Cohen, rising star in the domain of orthopedic surgery, currently in Philadelphia, Pennsylvania at the Jefferson University Health System. It was his vision that seemingly complex and complicated conditions of the musculoskeletal system can be simplified for an audience beyond orthopedic surgeons. He also believes that the knowledge and wisdom of experienced musculoskeletal surgeons can be passed along through a series of publications to the next generation of caregivers.

Painful conditions and physical impairments of the spine and extremities is a leading cause of morbidity and cost to our American society. The advances of biological science make the understanding of the functioning of the musculoskeletal system seem more difficult rather than simpler. This book is our attempt to bring the working knowledge of the foot and ankle into simple-to-understand concepts and explanations. If this book is to be successful, it will be because the information provided is understood by the reader, put to use when needed, and retained as a resource for the evaluation of people with foot and ankle conditions.

I

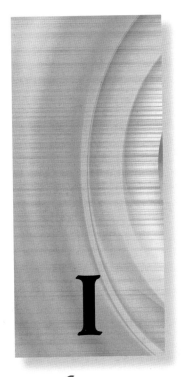

Physical Examination

1

Physical Examination of the Foot and Ankle

The Basics and Specific Tests

Ian Alexander, MD, FRCS(C)

Introduction

To be a useful diagnostic tool, the physical exam of any body part needs to be performed in a systematic manner to prevent critical omissions that come with a haphazard approach. This is certainly the case with the foot and ankle where, for example, immediately focusing on the painful part and neglecting to feel for pulses may lead to postoperative gangrene and subsequent limb amputation. In this chapter, we will outline a systematic approach to foot and ankle exam, that, with repeated performance, will make the reader a proficient clinical diagnostician.

Hurwitz SR, Parekh SG. *Musculoskeletal Examination of the Foot and Ankle: Making the Complex Simple* (pp. 2-26). © 2012 SLACK Incorporated.

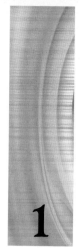

INSPECTION

Every musculoskeletal exam should start with inspection; however, the foot exam is a little different as it begins with assessment of the patient's footwear. Shoe upper deformation and sole wear can tell the astute observer a lot about the severity and chronicity of foot deformity or neuromuscular imbalance, especially if foot and ankle involvement is asymmetric. Additionally, the shoes a patient wears can tell you a lot about the patient's willingness to adapt to his or her condition and warn of unrealistic expectations in terms of treatment you might offer. Beware of almost any patient who comes to your office seeking relief of pain yet wears dress shoes that are much too small. The likelihood that surgical correction of the foot deformity will have a happy outcome is relatively low as these patients' expectations will be almost impossible to meet.

Step 1—Standing Inspection

Always ask your staff to have the patients remove their shoes, roll their pants up to their knees, and remain sitting in the chair. After completing your questioning, ask the patient to stand facing toward you. Standing inspection is essential, because many critical deformities will only be appreciated when the subject is weight bearing. Especially important to note in the standing patient are degree of hallux valgus and pronation; lesser toe deformity and, in particular, deviation between the second and third toes in comparison to the asymptomatic side; transverse plane forefoot position (forefoot abductus and adductus); and arch height. Then ask the patient to turn around and face away from you. In this position, note the alignment of the heel relative to the leg and look for abnormal visualization of digits laterally, the "too many toes" sign, a finding in pes planus with forefoot abductus. If the patient is flat footed, especially if this finding is unilateral, this is an appropriate time to do the single- and double-heel raise tests, the significance of which will be discussed in special tests for posterior tibial tendon dysfunction.

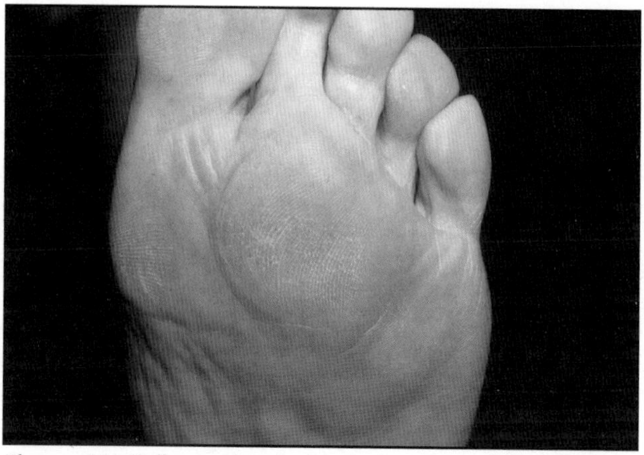

Figure 1-1. Callus under the second metatarsal head due to overload resulting from failed bunion surgery.

Step 2—Gait Assessment

Next the patient is asked to walk across the room and back. Although at normal walking speeds it is difficult to appreciate subtle gait abnormalities, avoidance patterns associated with hallux rigidus (no great toe extension after heel off), plantar fasciitis, heel pain syndrome or stress fracture (toe walking to avoid heel weight bearing), and external rotation gait with ankle arthrosis (to minimize anterior ankle impingement) are easily recognized if the symptoms are severe enough. Gait abnormalities may bring to light other orthopedic pathologies that may be directly or indirectly affecting the patient's foot complaints, such as knee arthritis, alternating foot loading, or back pathology that causes radicular foot pain.

Step 3—Sitting Inspection

With the patient in the sitting position, the examiner gets a closer look at the dorsal skin, but more importantly, the plantar aspect of the foot can be evaluated. Calluses on the plantar aspect of the foot can be indicative of mechanical overload or may be associated with plantar warts (Figure 1-1). These 2 conditions can be distinguished by the fact the warts can be multicentric and occur in non–weight-bearing areas, whereas calluses only occur where there is abnormal pressure or shear. On closer inspection, warts will typically have multiple tiny central black dots and a central core around which skin lines course. Calluses from pressure are simply thickened skin, and the skin lines pass straight through the lesion. Also characteristic of a wart is exquisite tenderness when the lesion is squeezed.

Plantar foot ulcers should be looked for, especially in diabetics with peripheral neuropathy, as they may not be appreciated by the patient with lack of sensation. Ulcers should be characterized as to location, dimensions, nature of the tissue in the base of the ulcer and that surrounds it, and whether the ulcer penetrates to the bone. To assess the latter, the ulcer should be probed with an instrument such as a hemostat. Obvious penetration to bone is usually indicative of osteomyelitis.

Palpation

It is an excellent habit to check the patient's pulses and assess sensation first as soon as you put your hands on the foot. When routine foot surgery leads to amputation related to postoperative gangrene or failed wound healing from poor circulation, failure of the surgeon to assess and record pulses preoperatively makes a legal defense difficult. The reasons for evaluating sensation in every case are 2-fold. First, nerve root irritation is a relatively common cause of foot pain, often without back or radicular symptoms. Second, patients with peripheral neuropathy frequently have problems healing osteotomies and arthrodeses, and it is surprising how often neuropathy precedes the diagnosis of type 2 diabetes mellitus. In addition, peripheral neuropathy itself can cause foot pain regardless of its etiology.

After assessing pulses and circulation, it is best to evaluate range of motion (ROM) of the critical articulations before palpating for tenderness, which, if severe, may result in guarding with voluntary apprehension-related loss of motion. Assessment of ankle, subtalar, and first and lesser metatarsophalangeal (MTP) motion will be discussed in the next section.

In most situations, the foot is being palpated for tenderness, but other significant findings on palpation include the presence of bony protuberances (usually juxta-articular osteophytes or exostosis resulting from soft tissue calcification), tendon or fascia-related pathology, and soft tissue masses. Percussion is an extension of palpation in which the examiner is looking for areas of nerve irritation or pathology and will be covered here as well.

Palpating for Tenderness

Accurately and knowledgeably palpating for tenderness is perhaps the most important diagnostic step in the physical exam. In essence, if you don't know your surface and related deep anatomy, you are not going to be a good diagnostician.

Articular Tenderness

Synovitis is what makes the joint line of articulations with pathology tender. It is also, in most cases, likely what makes these same joints painful when they are stressed at extremes of motion. At the extremes of motion, inflamed synovium is either being pinched and compressed or severely stretched. Since most foot articulations cross the long axis of the lower leg or foot, joint tenderness is invariably oriented in the coronal (midtarsal and MTP joints) or transverse (ankle) plane. Compared to other foot articulations, the subtalar joint is furthest from the surface. The sinus tarsi is the point at which inflamed subtalar synovium is most accessible to a palpating digit and tenderness here is frequent with subtalar pathology. Joint line tenderness is often accentuated by simultaneous stressing the joint to stretch the inflamed lining.

Tendon-Related Tenderness

Synovitis is also a likely contributor to the tenderness associated with tendinitis. In contrast to inflamed joints, the tenderness associated with tendon pathology is in the sagittal plane along the course of the tendon or at its insertion. Focal insertional tendinitis is most frequently seen with the Achilles tendon, the peroneus brevis, and the tibialis posterior. In addition, sesamoiditis can be caused by irritation at the insertion of the flexor hallucis brevis (FHB) at the proximal pole of the medial sesamoid. When tendon pathology is in the midsubstance, the tendon is often thickened, and the area of pathology is very tender. This tenderness is accentuated by resisted contraction of the

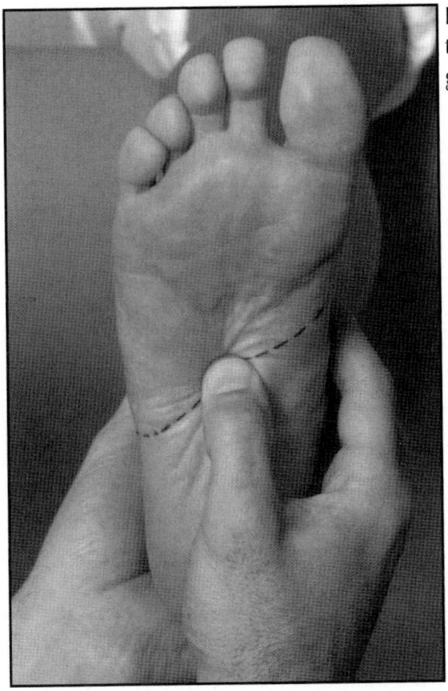

Figure 1-2. Path of maximum tenderness in peroneus longus tendinosis.

contiguous muscle. Without a doubt, knowledge of both a muscle's action and the course of its tendon is essential in making an accurate diagnosis. A good example of this is peroneus longus tendinosis in which tenderness is maximum in the plantar foot in a line between the cuboidal groove and first MT base with resisted first ray plantar flexion (Figure 1-2).

Fascia Tenderness

Enthesopathies like plantar fasciitis, in which tenderness is primarily localized to the plantar aspect of medial tubercle of the calcaneal tuberosity, are among the most common causes of foot pain. Extension of this tenderness to the medial aspect of the heel may be indicative of associated distal tarsal tunnel nerve entrapment, especially if associated with a positive percussion test.

Bone Tenderness

Bone tenderness is usually indicative of pathology. In the face of an acute injury, tenderness is frequently suggestive of fracture. In the presence of a fracture, ecchymosis and swelling are common, and acute deformity and bone crepitus diagnostic. Palpable deformity along a joint line may be due to a juxta-articular fracture or dislocation. Unrecognized juxta-articular fracture is a frequent cause of persistent pain after an ankle sprain. Evaluation of acute ankle sprain should include palpation of the areas where these missed fractures most often occur, including the base of the fifth metatarsal (MT), the anterior process of the calcaneus, the lateral process of the talus, the posterior margin of the lateral malleolus with a fibular avulsion with peroneal tendon dislocation, and lateral and posterior processes of the talus. Posterior process talar fractures are best loaded with forced ankle plantar flexion. Exquisite bone tenderness without an antecedent injury is suggestive of a stress or insufficiency fracture. Both of these are common in the lesser MT shafts, and stress fractures also occur in the navicular and calcaneus. Since most calcaneus fractures occur in the tuberosity in a line from just posterior to the posterior facet superiorly to a point just distal to the tubercles, inferiorly squeezing the heel between the thenar eminences of clasped hands (the heel squeeze test) will elicit exquisite tenderness in calcaneal stress fracture patients and mild to moderate discomfort in plantar fasciitis and heel pain syndrome patients (Figure 1-3).

Forefoot Tenderness

The location of maximum tenderness in patients with forefoot pain is very helpful in making an accurate diagnosis and prescribing the correct treatment. Many patients with metatarsalgia (pain in the forefoot) have associated tenderness plantar to the MT head. If limited to this area alone, the likely diagnosis is plantar capsulitis, a condition of the plantar plate analogous to rotator cuff tendinitis in the shoulder. This most often occurs in the second MTP. If it is associated with splaying of the second and third toes, second web space tenderness,

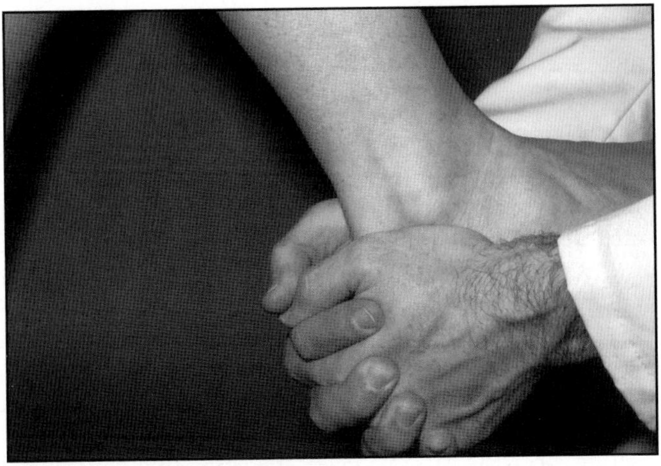

Figure 1-3. Heel squeeze test.

and/or a positive digital drawer test, a tear of the lateral capsule of the second MTP joint should be suspected. If plantar MTP joint tenderness is associated with dorsal joint line tenderness, there is likely synovitis of the MTP joint and possibly MT head avascular necrosis. If the tenderness is just plantar, extends proximal and distal to the joint, and is aggravated by resisted plantar flexion of the digit, flexor digitorum longus (FDL) tendinitis should be suspected as the cause of the forefoot pain. Tenderness isolated to the web space, especially the second and third, suggests the possibility of entrapment of the interdigital nerve and secondary neuroma. A complementary history of adjacent digit pain and numbness and findings of decreased web space sensation and a positive percussion sign support the neuroma diagnosis.

Nerve Tenderness

Nerves that are entrapped, surgically traumatized, embedded in surgical scar, or chronically irritated (eg, the medial plantar hallucal nerve in bunion patients) are very tender but more dramatically are sensitive to percussion with distal paresthesias resulting.

Palpable Bone Prominences and Soft Tissue Masses

Periarticular Osteophytes

Clinically significant periarticular osteophytes are common in the later stages of osteoarthrosis. They contribute to the limitation of joint motion and, when superficial, may cause painful skin irritation due to the friction from footwear. These symptomatic osteophytes are most common over the first MTP joint and the second and third tarsometatarsal joints where they are easily palpable. Ankle and subtalar osteophytes are deep and usually not palpable. A palpable osteophyte at the second MTP joint is almost diagnostic of second MT head avascular necrosis. In advanced stages of this condition the MT head collapses and flattens and bone is extruded dorsally forming a palpable ridge. Also virtually diagnostic of this late stage of second MT head avascular necrosis (AVN) is restricted dorsiflexion of the second toe at the MTP joint.

Other Bone Prominences

Other palpable bone prominences not related to a joint are unusual, but one that is occasionally seen is the "pump bump," a calcaneal exostosis that can be present just lateral to the Achilles tendon insertion and is felt to be related to chronic friction of footwear in the area. This problem is not uncommon in figure skaters whose boots rub in this region.

Soft Tissue Masses

Soft tissue masses of the foot are almost diagnostic when they occur in certain locations. Examples include the following:

- Achilles insertion: Painful swelling at the Achilles insertion is the hallmark of insertional Achilles tendinosis. Heterotopic calcification of the scarred tendon in this region is common.
- In substance Achilles tendon: Achilles tendinosis produces swelling in the Achilles tendon proximal to its insertion. The swelling is usually very hard and tender and often fusiform in line with the tendon.

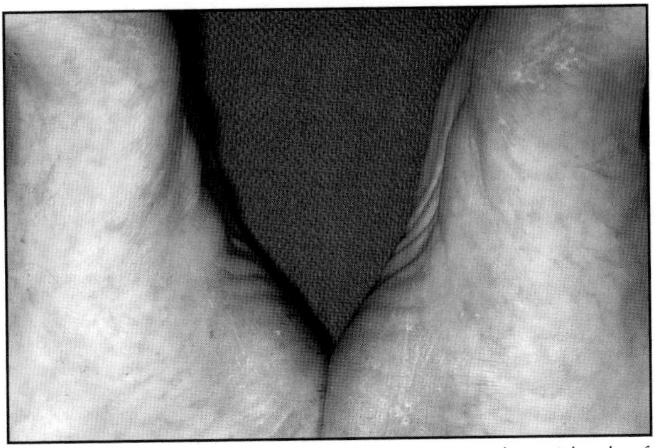

Figure 1-4. Nodules of plantar fibromatosis in the midarch of the left foot.

- Anteromedial ankle: A mass is seen in this location with rupture of the tibialis anterior as the tendon hangs up at the extensor retinaculum as it retracts.
- Mid arc: A nodule(s) less than 1 cm in diameter and embedded in the plantar fascia is characteristic of plantar fibromatosis, a fibrous tissue condition related to Dupuytren's contracture of the hand. Nodules may be multiple and closely spaced, but if an individual nodule exceeds 1 cm, concern about possible malignancy is appropriate (Figure 1-4).
- Web space: A mass may be palpable in interdigital neuroma, but in my experience this is unusual.
- Plantar pressure areas: Patients with rheumatoid arthritis frequently develop hard, generally mobile, subcutaneous nodules under the central heel and the first and fifth MT heads.

Range of Motion

Three lower leg joints are clinically important and their motion should be assessed with every foot and ankle evaluation. These are the first MTP joint, the ankle joint, and the subtalar joint complex, which includes the subtalar and talonavicular joints.

First Metatarsophalangeal Joint

The first MTP joint is important because 50% of toe weight bearing is through the hallux, and pathology of the first MTP joint contributes significantly to foot-related morbidity. Almost more important is that restricted painful motion of the first MTP joint can contribute significantly to other foot and ankle disorders. For example, the insidious onset of hallux rigidus can cause a gait pattern that completely avoids great toe weight bearing. This weight-bearing pattern over time causes repetitive stress to the tibialis posterior, which is called on with each step to maintain an inverted foot posture. If the examiner focuses on the patient's medial ankle pain and fails to recognize the first MTP pathology, surgical management of the patient's tibialis posterior tendon dysfunction without addressing the patient's hallux rigidus is almost certainly doomed to fail. The first MTP joint should be assessed with the ankle in relaxed plantar flexion, because most often the examiner is interested in restricted motion due to intra-articular pathology. If hallux plantar flexion is restricted in this position, a tight extensor hallucis longus (EHL) (often scarred from surgery) is suspected. If hallux dorsiflexion is restricted with the ankle neutral or in slight dorsiflexion, a contracted flexor hallucis longus (FHL) is suspected. This is a common finding in patients who habitually wear high-heeled shoes.

Ankle Joint

Ankle ROM can be assessed with 3 different leg positions. Most often ankle (sagittal) motion is assessed with the knee flexed and the foot relaxed. In certain situations, sagittal motion of the ankle should also be assessed with the foot held in neutral alignment and in others with the knee extended. In many cases, patients with chronic flatfoot deformities will have developed a gastrocsoleus contracture over time. In these patients, the foot fails to supinate at heel off, leaving the transverse tarsal joint (the talonavicular and calcaneocuboid joints) unlocked. In the unlocked position, forefoot dorsiflexion can occur through the transverse tarsal joint. Over time dorsiflexion at this level progressively reduces the need for ankle dorsiflexion. Progressive contracture of the gastrocsoleus further accentuates the situation. Assessment of the degree to which this has occurred is relatively simple: by supinating the forefoot and stabilizing the heel in neutral, the transverse tarsal joint is locked. With a tight gastrocsoleus and a locked midfoot there will be marked restriction of ankle dorsiflexion (often –30 degrees) when compared to the unlocked foot.

Ankle dorsiflexion should be assessed with the knee fully extended, especially in children with neurological conditions or those who are simply toe walkers. If ankle dorsiflexion is unrestricted with the knee flexed but severely restricted with the knee extended, this is indicative of a contracted gastrocnemius and a normal soleus as the gastroc crosses the knee joint and the soleus does not.

Subtalar Joint Complex

Normal coronal plane motion of the hindfoot is totally dependent on integrated intact function of both the subtalar and talonavicular joints. Restrict motion of either of these articulations and "subtalar motion" is lost. Assessing subtalar complex motion is difficult because it is easy to mistake coronal plane rocking of the talus in the ankle as subtalar motion. This is especially the case in individuals with chronic loss of subtalar motion, like talocalcaneal coalition, in which the ankle has compensated for a locked subtalar joint. The way to avoid this mistake is to palpate relative talar and calcaneal motion as the hindfoot is inverted and everted (Figure 1-5). This is accomplished by placing one index finger on the talus and the long finger on the calcaneus as the heel is moved and evaluating relative motion of the 2 fingers. If they move together, subtalar motion is absent. Similarly, talonavicular motion can be assessed by placing fingers on the navicular tuberosity and the medial talar head and assessing relative motion of the two as the foot is inverted and adducted and then everted and abducted.

Sensory Testing

Sensory Testing

All sensory testing should be done with a Semmes-Weinstein 5.07 monofilament (Zeus Inc, Orangeburg, South

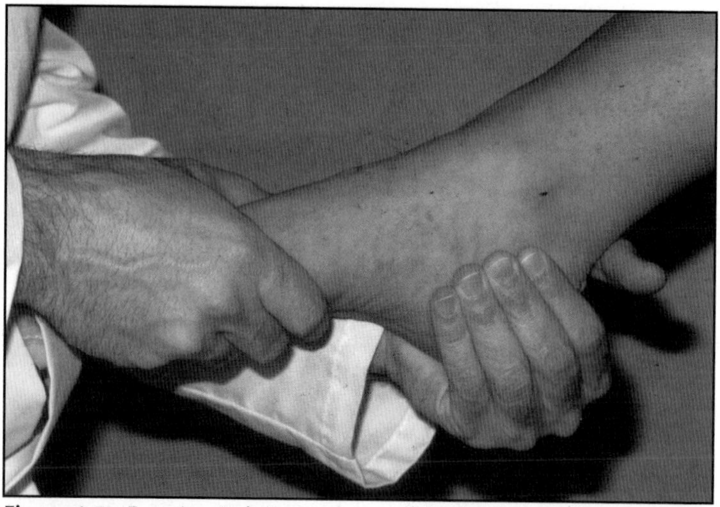

Figure 1-5. Examiner's digits on the medial subtalar joint line, manually assessing relative talocalcaneal motion as the foot is rocked into inversion and eversion.

Carolina). Perform the sensory exam as a routine immediately after assessing the pulses and this important portion of the exam is less likely to be forgotten. The areas of the foot checked will depend on the patient's presenting complaint. General screening is primarily for evidence of a nerve root lesion or peripheral neuropathy. With radicular symptoms, decreased sensation is usually in the lateral calf and dorsum of the foot (L5) or, less often, in the lateral border of the foot (S1). With neuropathy, the examiner tries to identify the level at which sensation decreases dramatically. Since medial lower leg sensation is generally intact, begin just below the medial knee joint line and check sensation to the medial malleolus. Next, start laterally just below the knee and check sensation to the lateral malleolus. Finally, check foot sensation from dorsomedial to lateral and then the plantar aspect of the foot. If the pain is in the forefoot, particularly if it radiates into 2 toes and is accompanied by numbness, comparative assessment of web space and plantar toe sensation is appropriate to help identify an interdigital neuroma. If the patient has a sprained ankle, always check anterolateral ankle and dorsolateral foot sensation because a tear of the intermediate dorsal cutaneous nerve, the lateral branch of the superficial peroneal nerve, can prolong disability associated with an ankle sprain. A similar area of numbness with or without a direct blow to the lateral lower leg may be indicative of superficial peroneal nerve entrapment where it passes through the lower leg fascia about 10 cm above the ankle and between 1 to 2 cm anterior to the fibular shaft. Heel pain associated with a decrease in plantar heel skin sensation suggests an associated problem with the medial calcaneal nerve either from prior heel surgery or entrapment at the fascial margin.

Decreased sensation over the medial aspect of the hallux can be associated with severe hallux valgus and secondary chronic nerve irritation or after bunion surgery where the nerve is embedded in scar tissue. In virtually all of these instances, the nerve at the point of entrapment or injury is tender and percussion will produce distal paresthesias.

Motor Exam

A motor exam is indicated when the patient's history or other exam findings suggest a neurological problem. Historical features that suggest a motor exam might be helpful include instability, giving way or tripping, muscle fatigue or weakness (especially with moderate levels of activity), radicular pain, and family history of a neurological disorder. Physical findings that indicate the need for a motor exam include gait abnormalities that are not simply due to pain, pes planus and pes cavus, and a positive sensory exam. In pain with radicular symptoms, weakness of the EHL is the most common finding. Peroneal weakness is common in these patients as well but is the hallmark of patients with a cavus foot on a neurological basis. Heel walking will bring out subtle weakness of the tibialis anterior. Difficulty toe walking or inability to perform repeated heel raises will be present in patients with gastrocsoleus weakness. This is difficult to identify on manual testing unless it is severe.

Specific Tests

Achilles Tendon Tears

Tears of the Achilles tendon are often missed for 3 reasons: 1) the inciting trauma is usually minimal as the injury occurs most often with either pushing off or simply running, 2) pain with complete tear can be fairly minimal, and 3) patients can remain remarkably functional, walking with a minimal limp even after complete disruption of the tendon. Patients with a complete rupture will have at least a mild limp. Swelling and bruising of the lower posterior calf is common. A palpable defect in the tendon about 4 to 5 cm above the calcaneal insertion is common. Other plantar flexors will often generate 5/5 power on manual muscle testing. The Thompson squeeze test is often helpful. With this test, the patient lies prone on a table or kneels on a chair. On the normal side, squeezing the resting calf muscle will produce ankle plantar flexion (Figure 1-6). On the affected side, squeezing the resting calf produces no ankle plantar flexion—a positive Thompson squeeze test (Figure 1-7).

Joint Instability

Whenever joint instability is assessed with manual manipulation maneuvers, it is mandatory to make a comparison to the contralateral "uninvolved side." Congenital ligamentous laxity can produce grossly positive instability tests, which are normal for a ligamentously lax individual. In these patients, findings on the "normal" side will be identical to those of the "abnormal." Two lower leg articulations are prone to ligamentous injury: the second MTP joint and the ankle.

Second Metatarsophalangeal Instability

Standing inspection gives you the first clue that second MTP instability may be a problem. Characteristically, the second MTP capsule is torn first on the lateral side. When the patient bears weight, the tendons crossing the joint become taut, and with a lateral capsular tear there is little resistance to medial drifting of the digit. This produces splaying of the second and third toes that is absent or minimal in the

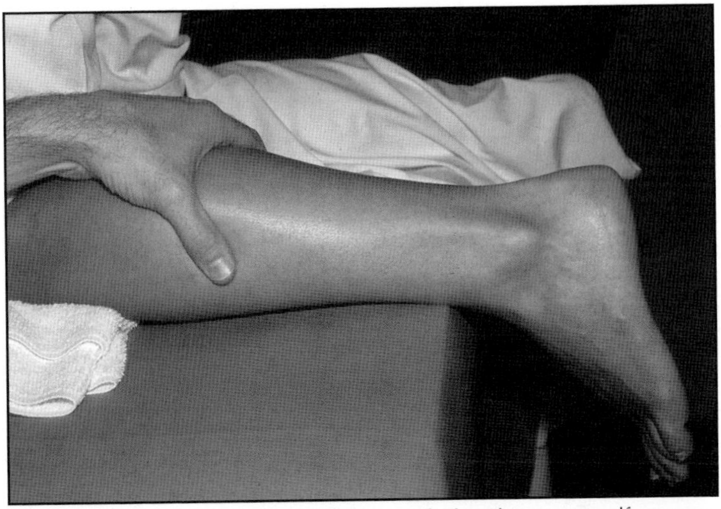

Figure 1-6. Normal foot plantar flexion with the Thompson calf squeeze test.

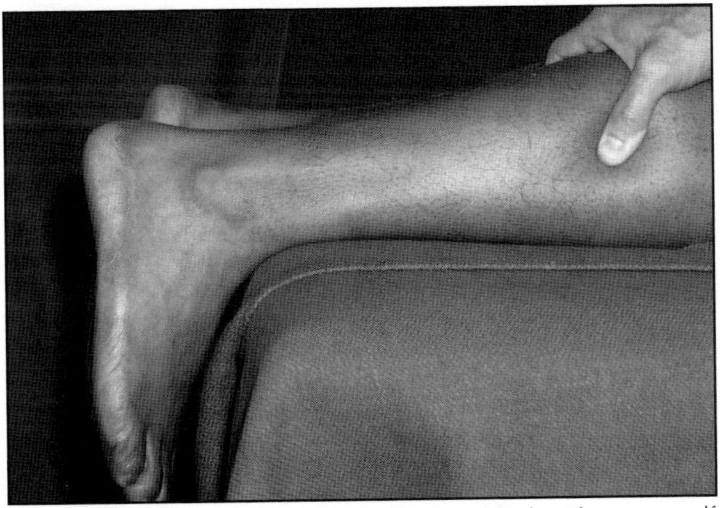

Figure 1-7. Absence of foot plantar flexion with the Thompson calf squeeze test due to a ruptured Achilles tendon (positive test).

non–weight-bearing foot (Figure 1-8). Even in the absence of this splaying, any patient complaining of forefoot pain, particularly if it is referable to the second MTP joint area, should have a digital drawer test to assess MTP stability. With this

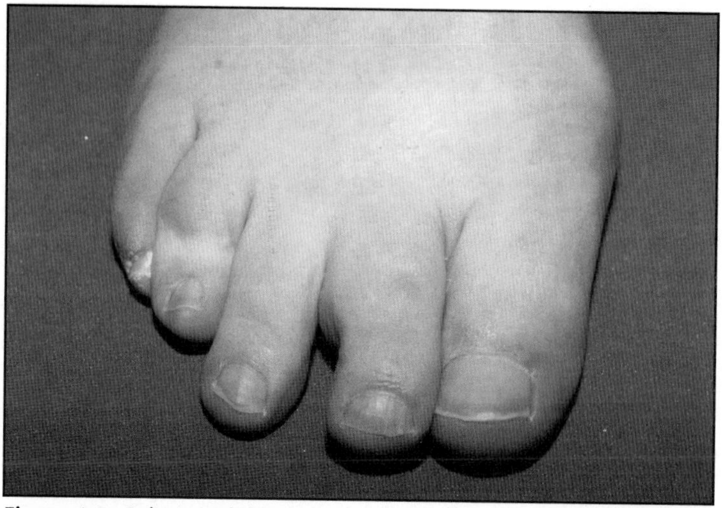

Figure 1-8. Splaying of the second and third toes in the presence of a second MTP joint capsular tear.

test, the examiner grasps the proximal phalanx between the index finger of the dominant hand over the dorsum of the neck and the thumb over the plantar base of the phalanx. The fingers of the nondominant hand grasp the second MT to stabilize the foot as the examiner presses upward on the base of the proximal phalanx (Figure 1-9). Normally the phalangeal base, relative to the MT head, will not subluxate or will move at most a couple of millimeters with a firm end point. Subluxation, as compared to the opposite side, can be graded as mild, moderate, or severe, and careful note should be made of any crepitus during the test. Occasionally, the toe will completely dislocate. If crepitus is present, it can be assumed that chronic subluxation or recurrent dislocation has resulted in severe abrasion or complete loss of dorsal MT head articular cartilage.

Ankle Instability

Manual testing of ankle instability is of questionable reliability. Even in individuals with a very reliable history of recurrent ankle instability, the anterior drawer test is usually negative. Most patients with a positive drawer sign will also have a positive drawer on the asymptomatic side, an indication that the positive drawer is probably more often a sign of

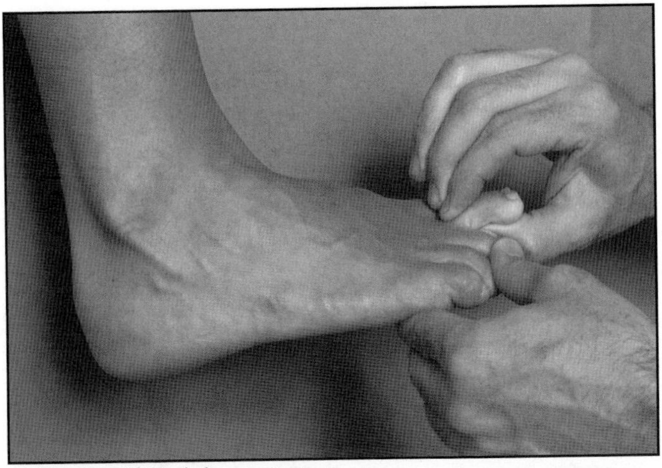

Figure 1-9. Digital drawer test.

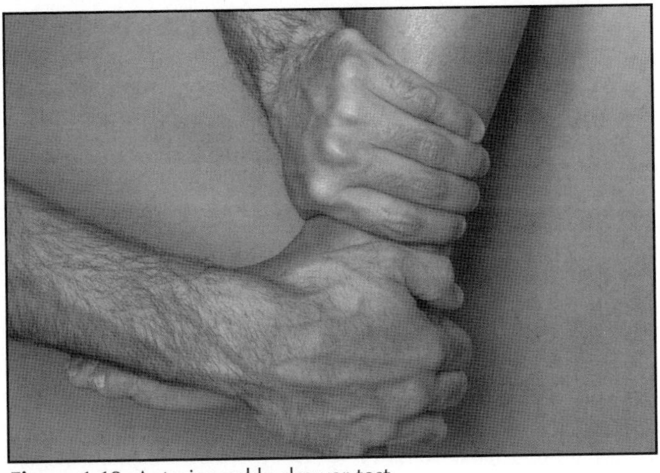

Figure 1-10. Anterior ankle drawer test.

generalized ligamentous laxity. In the acute setting, with post-traumatic pain, eliciting a positive anterior drawer sign is even less likely. The anterior drawer test is performed on a small patient by grasping the hindfoot (fingers around the heel and thumb over the talar neck) with the examiner's dominant hand and pushing the tibia posteriorly with the opposite hand. For larger patients, the dominant hand grasps the heel and the volar forearm wraps over the dorsum of the foot to block dorsiflexion as the foot is pulled forward (Figure 1-10).

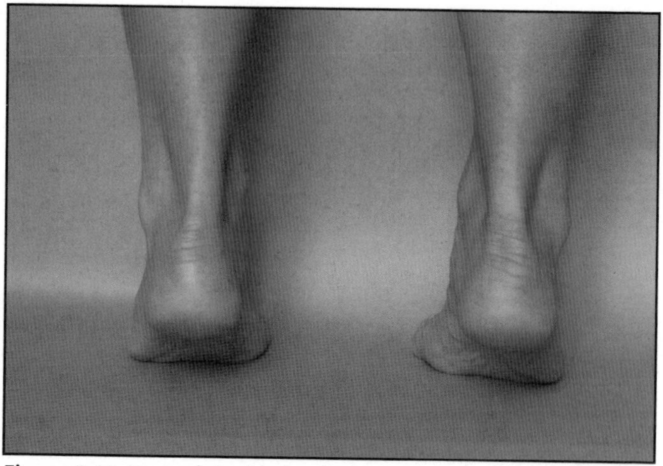

Figure 1-11. Normal double heel raise test.

Posterior Tibial Tendon Dysfunction

Tibialis posterior tendinosis can occur in young, especially flatfoot, patients. However, the syndrome of posterior tibial tendon dysfunction (PTTD) generally refers to middle aged or older patients that develop a progressive (usually unilateral) pes planus deformity after spontaneous onset of painful tibialis posterior tendinosis.

Stage I Posterior Tibial Tendon Dysfunction

In the early stages, the condition is characterized by medial ankle pain and swelling and a limp, but alignment is normal. Examination reveals boggy swelling along the tendon and marked tenderness. A discrete tendon may still be palpable with resisted inversion at this stage. The double heel raise is often normal, but the patient is usually unable to single heel raise (raise the heel while standing on one leg) due to pain. A normal double heel raise test means that with the patient standing facing a wall about a foot and a half away, with hands flat on the wall, the heels invert symmetrically when the patient is requested to go up on his or her toes (Figure 1-11).

Stage II Posterior Tibial Tendon Dysfunction

With progressive degeneration, attritional lengthening of the tendon occurs, and as a result, there is gradual flattening

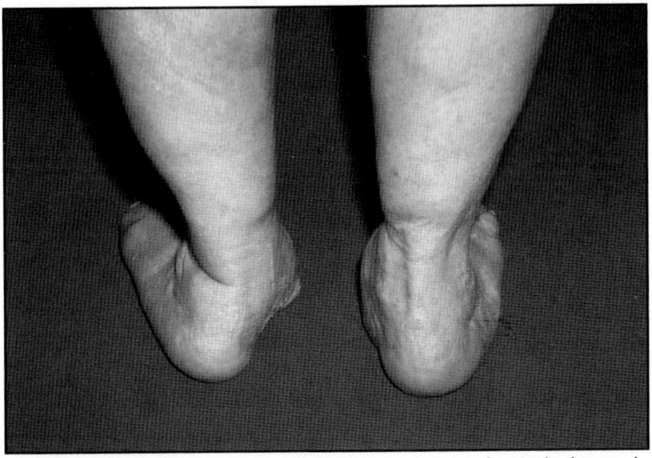

Figure 1-12. "Too many toes" sign in patient with rigid planovalgus foot and severe forefoot abductus.

of the longitudinal arch. With the double heel raise test, heel inversion is not symmetric. A discrete tendon is usually not palpable at this stage as the degenerative tendon is often thickened to many times its normal size. Once tendon elongation is severe or rupture complete, the heel will not invert at all on the double heel raise test. At this stage, ankle dorsiflexion should be assessed with the heel held inverted because patients, especially late stage II patients, will have a progressive contracture of the gastrocsoleus as dorsiflexion occurs through the transverse tarsal joint.

Stage III Posterior Tibial Tendon Dysfunction

In the late stages of PTTD, the arch is usually nonexistent, and there is often substantial associated forefoot abductus leading to what is described as the "too many toes" sign, where most of the lesser toes are visible lateral to the heel when inspecting the foot from the posterior (Figure 1-12). Characteristic of this stage is loss of subtalar joint complex mobility. A tight Achilles with a gastrocsoleus contracture is common.

Tarsal Tunnel Syndrome

Compression of the posterior tibial nerve and its branches in the tarsal tunnel is frequently discussed but not often seen. Tarsal tunnel syndrome is characterized by plantar foot numbness and, less often, pain. Decreased plantar sensation is present, and a positive percussion sign over the tarsal tunnel is essential. A mass in the tarsal canal may be the cause of the symptoms and should be sought with palpation. In my practice the most common cause of tarsal tunnel syndrome with a space-occupying lesion has been a protruding talocalcaneal coalition. This etiology should be suspected if subtalar motion is absent. Tarsal tunnel syndrome can also be associated with a pes planus deformity.

Interdigital Neuroma

The diagnosis of interdigital neuroma is completely dependent on history and physical exam. The complaints of a patient with interdigital neuroma are virtually diagnostic when they are classic. Classic complaints include the radiation of pain (often burning) and numbness of 2 adjacent toes, a need to remove constrictive shoes even when sitting, and a compulsion to vigorously massage the forefoot when the pain is severe. On physical exam no one sign is diagnostic, but a combination of positive clinical signs is highly suggestive. These include single web space tenderness, single web space decreased sensation, a positive percussion test over just the involved interdigital nerve, a palpable mass (rare), and a positive Mulder's click, which is a palpable click that occurs when the forefoot is squeezed in the transverse plane. In some cases, this will produce paresthesias radiating into the patient's affected toes.

Cavovarus Foot

The primary deformity in most cavovarus feet is a plantarflexed first ray. This creates the appearance of a high arch and a forefoot valgus that must be compensated by hindfoot varus in midstance. Plantar flexion of the first ray in Charcot-Marie-Tooth (CMT) disease is due to muscle imbalance with relative overpull of the peroneus longus compared to its weak antagonist, the tibialis anterior. In CMT, hindfoot varus is aggravated by a weak peroneus brevis that fails to exert its normal control of hindfoot inversion in midstance.

All steps of the exam previously outlined are critical in planning therapy for patients with a symptomatic cavovarus foot. Standing inspection reveals a high arch foot with a varus heel and forefoot adductus. In these patients, determining the rigidity of the deformity is important in planning treatment. Helpful in this regard is the Coleman lateral block test. A series of blocks of wood are placed under the patient's heel and lateral forefoot, allowing the first MT head to rest on the floor. This test posts the forefoot laterally, eliminating the need for compensatory hindfoot varus that is usually brought on by the forefoot valgus and the tripod effect (the need to get the first and fifth MTs and the heel to the ground at foot flat). With the laterally placed block in the Coleman test, a flexible hindfoot varus will be reduced to neutral (Figure 1-13). If the hindfoot varus is fixed, correction will not occur with the Coleman lateral block test (Figure 1-14).

Sensory and motor testing are critical in these patients, as in the late stages many will have a significant sensory neuropathy and identifying which muscles are weak is important in surgical treatment. Assessing specific joint ROM as previously outlined is also critical because in the later stages, fixed ankle equinus, or at least limited ankle dorsiflexion, is common and must be addressed if surgery is elected. Assessing the rigidity of first ray plantar flexion is also important as a dorsiflexion osteotomy of the first MT and, in many cases, the second and third MTs, is often performed. To do this, the first MT head is grasped between the thumb (plantar) and index finger of one hand and the second MT head by the thumb and index finger of the other. With the second MT head held stationary, the first MT head is translated up and down. The alignment of the 2 thumb nails is observed. Normally there is approximately 1 cm of dorsal and 1 cm of plantar translation of the first MT head compared to the second. In the planus foot there is hypermobility, and dorsal translation will be 2 cm and plantar translation 0 to 1 cm. In the cavus foot, the first ray is stiff and plantarflexed and dorsal translation will be 0 or even negative in severe cases, and plantar translation 1 cm, and occasionally 2 cm (Figure 1-15). Examination of the patient with a cavus foot in the prone position is also advisable. In this position with the talonavicular joint reduced, measurement of the center line of the heel is made to the center line of the calf and, subsequently, the center line of the heel to the transverse plane of the forefoot. These measurements will give

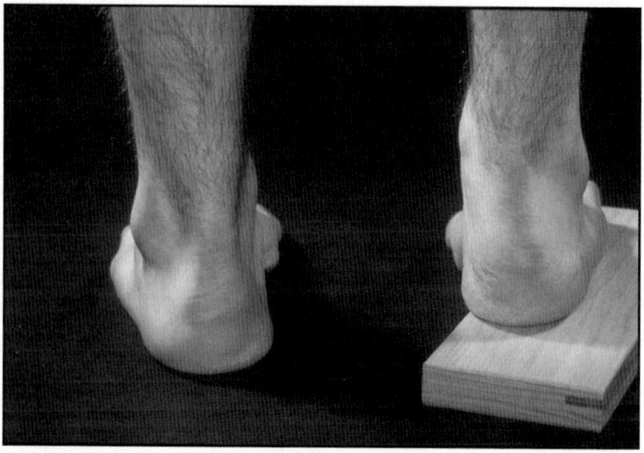

Figure 1-13. Normal Coleman lateral block test. Hindfoot varus corrects with the block in place

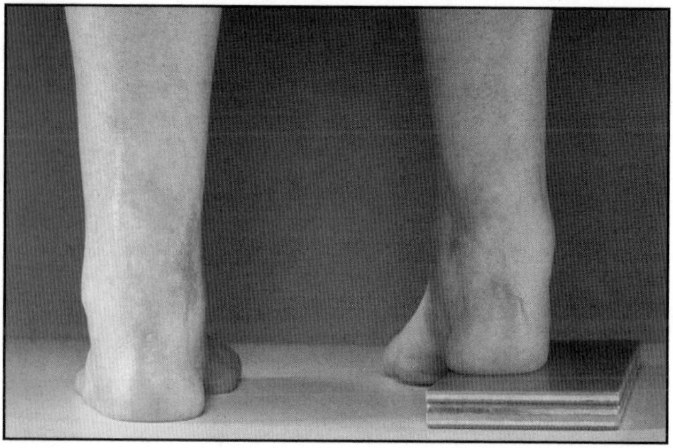

Figure 1-14. Abnormal Coleman lateral block test. Hindfoot varus does not correct with the block in place, indicating rigid hindfoot varus.

the examiner an idea of the degree of fixed hindfoot varus and the severity of forefoot valgus, which are helpful in planning orthotic and surgical correction (Figure 1-16).

2

Gait Analysis and Clinical Relevance

Sudheer Reddy, MD

Introduction

Evaluation of the foot and ankle as it relates to gait is a complex phenomenon. However, its proper functioning is essential to normal gait. Disorders of the foot and ankle, as a result, often result in a disruption of gait and locomotion. It is important, therefore, for the clinician to understand how to evaluate both normal and pathologic gait.

There are 6 basic determinants of gait as defined by Saunders et al: 1) pelvic rotation, 2) pelvic obliquity, 3) knee flexion in stance, 4) foot and ankle motion, 5) lateral displacement of the pelvis, and 6) axial rotations of the lower extremities.[1] Abnormalities of 2 or more of these determinants can

Hurwitz SR, Parekh SG. *Musculoskeletal Examination of the Foot and Ankle: Making the Complex Simple* (pp. 27-36). © 2012 SLACK Incorporated.

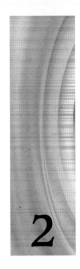

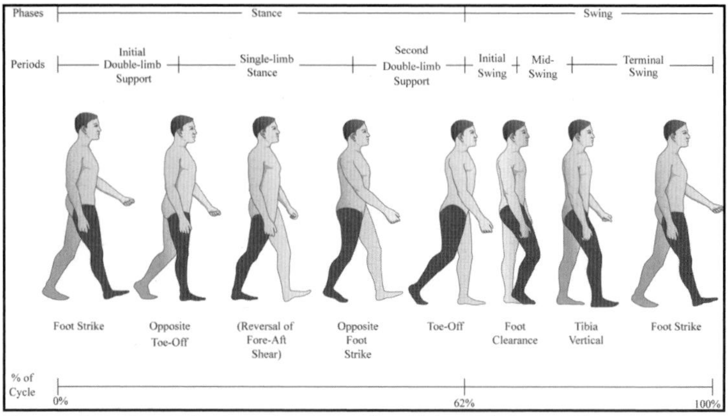

Figure 2-1. Typical normal gait cycle. (Adapted from Chambers HG, Sutherland DH. A practical guide to gait analysis. *J Am Acad Orthop Surg.* 2002;10:222-231.)

lead to inefficient gait or pathologic gait.[1,2] In particular, disorders of the foot and ankle affect both foot and ankle motion and axial rotations of the lower extremities.

There are 5 prerequisites of normal gait: 1) stability of the weight-bearing foot throughout the stance phase, 2) clearance of the non–weight-bearing foot during swing phase, 3) appropriate prepositioning during terminal swing of the foot for the next gait cycle, 4) adequate step length, and 5) energy conservation.[3] Pathologic states of the foot and ankle can affect each of these prerequisites and thus affect gait overall.

Gait Cycle: Periods and Functions

The gait cycle is typically divided into 8 distinct parts that define the functional periods and phases of the cycle: 1) foot strike, 2) opposite toe-off, 3) reversal of fore shear to aft shear, 4) opposite foot strike, 5) toe-off, 6) foot clearance, 7) tibia vertical, and 8) foot strike (Figure 2-1).[3] Terms such as *heel strike* have been used to describe gait but should be avoided as these specific events could be absent or altered in individuals with a pathologic gait.[3]

Table 2-1

GAIT CYCLE: TIMING AND FUNCTIONS

Interval	*Percent of Gait Cycle (Range)*	*Function*	*Opposite (Contralateral) Limb*
Initial foot contact—double-limb support	0 to 15	Weight acceptance	Preparing for swing (preswing)
Single-limb stance	15 to 50	Balanced support of entire body	Swing
Second double-limb support	50 to 65	Preparation for swing (preswing)	Weight acceptance
Initial swing	65 to 75	Foot clearance for swing leg	Single-limb stance (support of entire body)
Midswing	75 to 85	Advancement of swing limb	Single-limb stance
Terminal swing	85 to 100	Swing limb deceleration	Single-limb stance

Adapted from Chambers HG. A practical guide to gait analysis. *J Am Acad Orthop Surg.* 2002;10:222-231.

Stance phase occurs when the foot is in contact with the ground from foot strike to toe-off and constitutes approximately 60% of the gait cycle (Table 2-1). The stance phase itself is divided into 3 distinct periods: 1) initial double-limb support (loading response), 2) single-limb stance, and 3) second double-limb support (preswing). Of note, the cardinal events for initial double-limb support are foot strike and opposite toe-off while the defining events for single-limb stance are opposite toe-off and opposite foot strike.[3] During the gait cycle, the foot changes from a flexible structure at foot strike to a rigid structure at toe-off. The ankle joint functions as a mitered hinge since upon foot strike there is internal tibial rotation, hindfoot eversion, and a supple transverse tarsal (Chopart's joint, which includes the talonavicular and calcaneocuboid joints). Internal rotation of the tibia allows the transverse tarsal joints to unlock, allowing both the hindfoot and leg to absorb the impact of foot strike. When foot strike occurs, the anterior muscles undergo eccentric joint contraction to control progression from foot strike to foot flat to absorb energy and stabilize the foot.[3,4] During foot strike, the foot is pronated to unlock Chopart's joint. This allows for a flexible midfoot that allows the foot to accept weight transfer during the transition from the foot strike to the foot flat stage. The foot is pronated as a result of internal rotation of the tibia and subsequent hindfoot valgus (hindfoot eversion). The tibialis posterior acts at the foot flat stage to prevent overpronation.[3,4] During the foot flat stage, the leg externally rotates along with midfoot supination and hindfoot inversion. The latter is accomplished by the action of the tibialis posterior, which initiates subtalar inversion. These actions then create a rigid transverse tarsal joint that allows the foot to serve as a platform for toe-off.[3] At the end of the foot flat stage, the tibialis posterior and gastrocnemius-soleus complex are activated to effect heel rise. Of note, the supination of the foot during the transition from foot flat to toe-off is accomplished by both the external rotation of the leg and also by the windlass mechanism. The windlass mechanism is the tension placed on the plantar fascia as a result of dorsiflexion of the foot that increases the midfoot arch height and locks the transverse tarsal joint.[3,5-7]

Swing phase occurs when foot is off the ground from toe-off to the next heel strike and constitutes 38% of the cycle.[3] The swing phase is also divided into 3 stages: 1) initial swing, 2) midswing, and 3) terminal swing, with the defining events for initial swing being toe-off and foot clearance and terminal swing beginning with tibia vertical and being completed with foot strike.[3]

Additional terminology that must be understood when analyzing gait are gait velocity, step length, and stride length. Gait velocity is defined in units of cm/s or m/min or cadence (number of steps/min). The step length is the distance from the foot strike of one foot to the foot strike of the contralateral foot, while the stride length is the distance from the foot strike of one foot to the foot strike of the ipsilateral foot.[3]

In characterizing the gait pattern of an individual, it is important to understand 2 critical components of gait: 1) characterization of the dynamic muscular control of the foot and ankle (seen on the electromyographic [EMG] report), and 2) understanding the result of the sequential muscle activities on the mechanical characteristics of the foot and ankle during the gait cycle.[3] Of note, the ground reaction force during walking reaches approximately 1.5 times body weight. In comparison, running, in which there is a float phase when neither limb is on the ground, generates approximately 3 times body weight.[3]

Clinical Evaluation

Proper gait analysis should always start with a thorough physical examination of the entire lower extremity. The range of motion of the hips, knees, and ankles and subtalar joints should be documented. Particular attention should be given to contractures, deformities, and prior injuries that can affect gait. In regard to joint motion at the foot and ankle, ankle dorsiflexion is 20 degrees while plantar flexion is 40 degrees. Subtalar inversion and eversion are 25 degrees and 5 degrees, respectively. Subtalar motion is accomplished primarily at the transverse tarsal joints. Forefoot adduction is approximately 20 degrees, while abduction is 10 degrees. The metatarsophalangeal (MTP) joints should also be assessed, with the first MTP joint allowing approximately 45 degrees of flexion and 70 to 90 degrees of extension. The MTP joints should be tested for swelling, tenderness, or limitation of motion. Of note, while standing, deviation of the second or third toe can indicate lateral collateral ligament or plantar plate insufficiency.

A proper neuromuscular exam should also be conducted to evaluate for any subtle neuromuscular imbalance that can lead to gait pathology. Testing of the tibialis anterior involves asking the patient to walk on his or her heels. To manually test this muscle, have the patient forcibly dorsiflex and invert the foot. The tibialis anterior is predominantly innervated by L4. Testing of the extensor hallucis longus should involve forcible dorsiflexion of the great toe and is predominantly innervated by L5. Testing of the extensor digitorum longus (EDL) also involves having the patient walk on his or her heels, and to manually test this muscle, one should have the patient forcibly dorsiflex the toes. It is innervated by L5. This maneuver will also test extensor digitorum brevis (EDB) (although it cannot be isolated for manual muscle testing). Testing of the peroneus longus and brevis should be accomplished by securing the ankle by stabilizing the calcaneus and having the patient plantarflex and evert the foot against resistance. These 2 muscles are innervated by S1. Testing of the gastrocnemius-soleus complex should commence with asking the patient to walk on his or her heels and then asking the patient to jump up and down on the first MTP joints of the feet (balls of feet) one foot at a time. Manual muscle testing of this complex is difficult since it is stronger than all other leg muscles, making it difficult to detect existing muscle weakness.[8] Manual testing of the flexor hallucis longus (FHL) should occur by having the patient forcibly flex the hallux against resistance. Testing of the flexor digitorum longus (FDL) should occur by the same fashion with the patient flexing the toes against resistance.

Second, the patient should be observed walking both away from and toward the examiner. The clinician should pay particular attention to pelvic tilt if present; duration of stance and stride phases; range of motion at the hip, knee, and ankle; and use of assistive devices if any. The patient should also be asked to walk in tandem (with one foot directly in front of the other). Difficulty with tandem gait can reveal problems with balance and proprioception.[9] As an example, patients who have undergone an ankle fusion can have a decreased stance phase of gait as the loss of motion leads to a disruption of the normal progression from foot strike to toe-off.[10] Another example is that of a steppage gait, in which the affected limb is lifted higher to allow for adequate ground clearance of the foot. This is due to weakness of the musculature of the anterior compartment of the leg.[8] It is important also when evaluating gait to understand the difference between kinetics and kinematics. Kinetics involves the effect of forces on the motion of bodies while kinematics describes the motion of bodies regardless of the effects of force or mass.[8]

It is also important to realize that the gait of an individual changes with age. In particular, a shorter, broader-based stride is utilized with an approximately 10% to 20% decrease in gait velocity. Elderly males tend to walk with a flexed posture as well. While many gait disturbances in the elderly are found to be multifactorial and nonspecific, it is important to systematically examine the gait patterns of elderly individuals.[9]

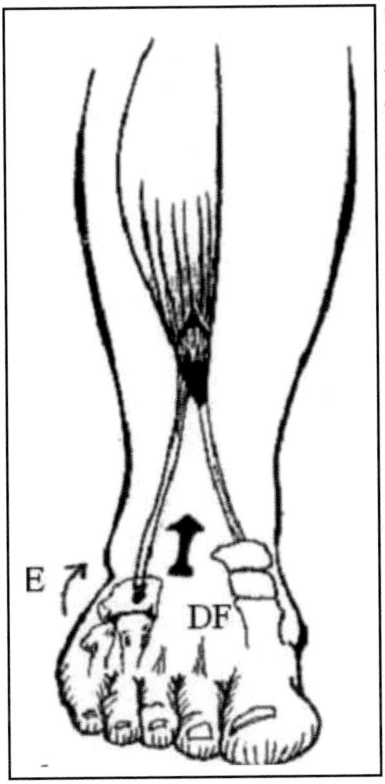

Figure 2-2. Diagram of split anterior tibial tendon transfer (SPLATT) for an equinovarus foot (E = eversion force; DF = dorsiflexion force). (With kind permission from Springer Science+Business Media: *Clin Orthop.* Fixation techniques for split anterior tibialis transfer in spastic equinovarus feet. 466, 2008, Hosalkar HS, Goebel J, Reddy S, Pandya NK, Keenan MA.)

Laboratory Evaluation

Observation of gait is important since it gives the clinician clues about what specific disorder or disorders are present and how they impact gait. However, formal gait analysis in a laboratory setting is important to elucidate the biomechanical basis for a pathologic gait. Laboratory evaluation of gait involves the use of EMG to evaluate muscle activity, force plate data analysis, 3-dimensional movements, kinetic and kinematic analysis, and energetics to fully evaluate a pathologic gait. As an example, EMG analysis could reveal swing phase spasticity of the tibialis anterior resulting in an inability to clear the swing phase limb. This spasticity could be addressed with an ankle-foot orthosis or surgically via a split anterior tibial tendon transfer (Figure 2-2).[11]

Kinematic data during gait analysis are obtained via skin markers that are placed on the patient's body. The position of these markers is captured serially by cameras as the patient walks down a walkway. Positional information as well as joint motion can be obtained by the data recorded. These data can then be processed in a 3-dimensional fashion and also compared to prior gait analyses as well as standard gait patterns for a specific age group. Information regarding loss or excessive joint motion can be derived. Kinetic data pertain to the forces acting on a body at any one time. It relates to the muscles that are contracting at any point in time, ground reaction forces, the patient's center of mass, and the center of rotation of each joint. These data are obtained from force plates on which the patient walks during the gait analysis.[3] The force plates are set so that as the patient ambulates, the transducers obtain information regarding gait velocity, medial-lateral shear of the foot during ambulation, vertical force, and torque with each step. These values can then be compared to the contralateral side and also to normal values for the particular patient's age group. Internal and external moments with respect to the joint are also reported. Internal moments are forces acting on a joint secondary to muscle contraction while external moments are forces experienced by a joint due to the ground reaction force. The 3-dimensional kinetic information obtained is clinically useful in evaluating the optimal prosthesis for amputees, joint contractures, the need for tendon transfers or releases, and shoes or orthotics.

Muscle activity is another parameter that is evaluated during gait analysis. It is difficult from observation only to determine whether a particular muscle is active at a particular point in time of the gait cycle. As a result, surface EMG electrodes are utilized to help determine which muscles are active and level of activity demonstrated during each point in time of the gait cycle. For superficial muscle groups, such as the adductors or quadriceps, surface electrodes are utilized to determine activity. For muscles that are deeper, fine wire EMG electrodes are utilized to obtain information on muscle activity. When the EMG data are combined with the kinetic and kinematic data, the clinician has a better understanding of the pattern of a particular individual's gait.

Foot pressure measurements are also obtained during gait analysis and are helpful in planning surgical intervention or orthotic prescriptions. There are 2 main types of methods of obtaining foot pressure measurements. The first is by placing foot pressure transducers into an individual's shoe, and the second is by having the patient walk on a force plate transducer. As an example, a cavus foot due to Charcot-Marie-Tooth disease can reveal excess pressure at the first metatarsal head and also along the lateral border of the foot due to hindfoot varus. This information can be used in orthotic fitting (lateral heel wedge and lateral post) or in planning surgical intervention such as a dorsiflexion osteotomy of the first metatarsal and a lateral closing wedge osteotomy of the calcaneus if surgery is required to correct the deformity. Furthermore, foot pressure measurements can also be used postoperatively to determine to what degree the intervention has improved the balance of the foot.[3,5,8]

Energetics is the final parameter that is often obtained during formal gait analysis. It is particularly important in evaluating amputees who expend more energy with ambulation. Energetics is simply the measurement of energy expenditure. One of the goals of achieving an optimal gait pattern is to reduce the amount of energy expended in daily ambulation. Energy expenditure can be obtained in 1 of 3 ways: 1) measurement of O_2 or CO_2 expenditure during ambulation, 2) measurement of the patient's pulse once a steady state has been achieved following ambulation, and 3) use of force plates during ambulation to calculate the amount of work that has been performed during ambulation, which can be used to determine how much energy is being expended. Each method has its disadvantages and advantages. As an example, measuring expired CO_2 requires the patient to wear a breathing apparatus while ambulating and the fact that oxygen consumption can vary during the day.[3,8] Measurement of the patient's pulse is the least invasive but is also the least precise.

Conclusion

Normal gait is the cyclical weight acceptance and swing phases of the bipedal mode in which humans walk. Abnormal gait is a sign and possibly a symptom of an abnormality in the neuromusculoskeletal apparatus. Normal gait reflects a pain-free and energy-efficient use of the trunk and lower extremities in walking. Gait analysis is a means of measuring motion of limb segments, calculating muscle and joint forces, and determining the oxygen consumption (energy expenditure) in moving forward along the ground. There is great importance to the foot and ankle function during stance and gait since it is the foot that contacts the ground and initiates a gait cycle. The measurements provided by gait analysis hold great promise in analyzing mechanisms of dysfunction in walking and assisting the clinician in determining underlying causes of gait abnormality, be it a foot, knee, limb length, or hip problem. Gait analysis may start with simple visual observation aided by video recordings that can be slowed to aid in diagnosis. The ultimate aim of gait analysis is to provide the patient with an effective treatment for gait disturbance via physical modalities, bracing, medication, or surgery.

References

1. Saunders JB, Inman VT, Eberhart HD. The major determinants in normal and pathological gait. *J Bone Joint Surg Am.* 1953;35-A(3):543-558.
2. Anderson FC, Pandy MG. Individual muscle contributions to support in normal walking. *Gait Posture.* 2003;17(2):159-169.
3. Chambers HG, Sutherland DH. A practical guide to gait analysis. *J Am Acad Orthop Surg.* 2002;10(3):222-231.
4. Gage JR, DeLuca PA, Renshaw TS. Gait analysis: Principle and applications with emphasis on its use in cerebral palsy. *Instru Course Lect.* 1996;45:491-507.
5. Perry J. *Gait Analysis: Normal and Pathological Function.* Thorofare, NJ: SLACK Incorporated; 1992.
6. Thordarson DSH, Schmotzer H, Chon J, Peters J. Dynamic support of the human longitudinal arch. A biomechanical evaluation. *Clin Orthop Relat Res.* 1995;316:165-172.
7. Huang CK, Kitaoka HB, An KN, Chao EY. Biomechanical evaluation of longitudinal arch stability. *Foot Ankle.* 1993;14(6):353-357.
8. Chiodo C, Bluman EM. Biomechanics of the Foot and Ankle. In: Pinzur M, ed. *Orthopaedic Knowledge Update 4: Foot and Ankle.* Rosemount, IL: American Academy of Orthopaedic Surgeons; 2008:3–13.
9. Lim MR, Huang RC, Wu A, Girardi FP, Cammisa FP. Evaluation of the elderly patient with an abnormal gait. *J Am Acad Orthop Surg.* 2007;15(2):107-117.
10. Thomas R, Daniels TR, Parker K. Gait analysis and functional outcomes following ankle arthrodesis for isolated ankle arthritis. *J Bone Joint Surg Am.* 2006;88:526-535.
11. Hosalkar HS, Goebel J, Reddy S, Pandya NK, Keenan MA. Fixation techniques for split anterior tibialis transfer in spastic equinovarus feet. *Clin Orthop Relat Res.* 2008;466(10):2500-2506.

II

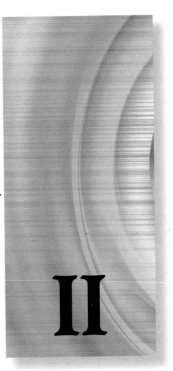

General Imaging

3

General Imaging of the Adult Foot and Ankle

David I. Pedowitz, MD

Introduction

Continued technological advances in diagnostic imaging have vastly improved our ability to accurately diagnose orthopedic pathology of the foot and ankle. Additionally, the availability of these tools at even some of the most remote practice locations allows us to appropriately plan the proper interventions for complex problems that were once routinely relegated to tertiary centers where advanced imaging was possible. Developing a sound understanding of the roles that these different modalities can play is essential if one is to render accurate and cost-efficient diagnostic services.

Hurwitz SR, Parekh SG. *Musculoskeletal Examination of the Foot and Ankle: Making the Complex Simple* (pp. 38-57). © 2012 SLACK Incorporated.

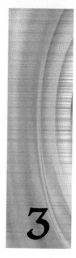

Plain Radiography

The cornerstone of diagnostic imaging, and the modality with which we are most familiar, is the plain radiograph. Routine radiography is often employed at initial patient evaluations in the outpatient setting or in the emergency room because it provides an outstanding screening tool for many foot and ankle conditions. Limitations include variability in patient body habitus, positioning and beam distance, beam strength, and the degree of penetration.

It is generally felt that all thorough initial patient evaluations of foot and ankle complaints should include plain radiographs. When trauma is involved, the Ottawa Ankle Rules provide guidelines as to those cases in which an x-ray should certainly be obtained (Table 3-1).[1] Standard views of the foot and ankle should be obtained weight bearing, unless clinically contraindicated, to help assess dynamic and degenerative pathology that might not be evident on non–weight-bearing films. The exact process of obtaining the standard views including film and beam placement is beyond the scope of this text and one should be referred to a comprehensive radiology or orthopedic foot and ankle text for how to perform these examinations.

Plain Radiography of the Foot

Traditional views include an anteroposterior (AP), lateral, and oblique projection of the foot. One must take time to familiarize oneself with the normal overlap of tarsal bones and their relationships. Keep in mind that there are 2 arches in the foot: a longitudinal arch seen on a lateral radiograph and a transverse arch in the coronal plane. It is the combination of these arches that accounts for tremendous overlap of the bones in the foot on plain radiographs. If one fails to realize these peculiar relationships in advance, recognizing midfoot and tarsal pathology becomes very difficult. When subtle pathology is suspected, contralateral films can provide a useful comparison.

Subtle features to note on foot radiographs are listed below. This is by no means an exhaustive list but should serve as an introduction to important and commonly used measurements and features of these studies.

Table 3-1

Ottawa Ankle Rules

X-rays of the ankle should be obtained if there is:

- Bony tenderness along the distal 6 cm of the posterior edge of the tibia or tip of the medial malleolus
- Bony tenderness along the distal 6 cm of the posterior edge of the fibula or tip of the lateral malleolus
- Inability to bear weight both immediately following the injury and then for 4 steps in the emergency department

Ottawa Foot Rules

Radiographs are indicated if there is bony pain in the mid-foot zone and any one of the following:

- Bony tenderness at the base of the fifth metatarsal
- Bony tenderness at the navicular bone
- Inability to bear weight both immediately following the injury and then for 4 steps in the emergency department

Exclusions: pregnancy and those with diminished ability to follow the test (eg, due to head injury or intoxication).

Adapted from Stiell IG, Greenberg GH, McKnight RD, Nair RC, McDowell I, Worthington JR. A study to develop clinical decision rules for the use of radiography in acute ankle injuries. *Ann Emerg Med.* 1992;21(4):384-390.

AP projection (Figure 3-1A) shows the following:

1. Relationships of sesamoids to first metatarsal (MT) head—normally directly underneath the first MT head—may appear lateralized in hallux valgus.
2. Bipartite sesamoids.
3. Additional accessory bones: Sesamoids in the flexor tendons to the lesser toes may be visualized at the level of the metatarsophalangeal joints (MTPJs).
4. Accessory navicular may be obscured by the large navicular tuberosity.
5. Os peroneum is a sesamoid bone located within the peroneus longus tendon. Typically located at the level of the cuboid. Proximal retraction can indicate rupture.

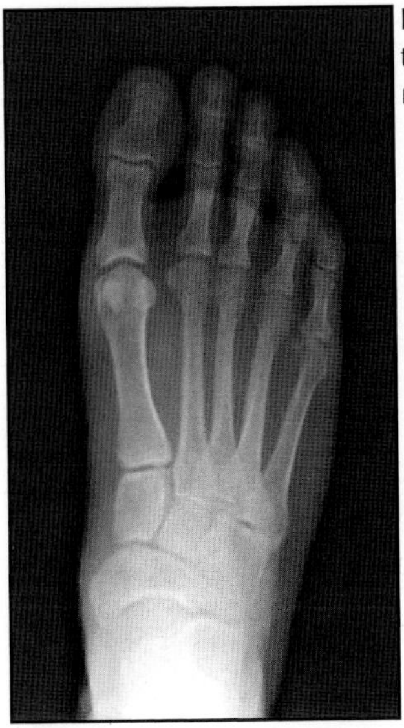

Figure 3-1A. Weight-bearing AP view of the foot. Note rare sesamoids beneath metatarsal heads 2 and 5.

6. The medial aspect of the second MT base should line up with the medial aspect of the middle cuneiform. Failure to maintain this relationship suggests injury to the "Lisfranc's ligament," which spans between the medial cuneiform and the base of the second MT.
7. Look for overlap and complete obscurity of joint space at the proximal interphalangeal joints of toes 2 to 4, which is typical in a flexion deformity at that joint (hammer toe).
8. Loss of joint space and overlap of the base of the proximal phalanx at the MTPJ is consistent with subluxation or a fixed deformity at this joint (clawing).
9. Degenerative changes at the first MTPJ are manifested by loss of joint space, osteophytes, and subchondral sclerosis.
10. Hallux valgus angle: Angle formed between a line drawn down the long axis of the proximal phalanx of the hallux and one drawn along the long axis of the first MT (normal <15 degrees). A larger angle signifies hallux valgus while a small or negative angle indicates hallux varus.
11. Accessory bones and atypical sesamoid bones.

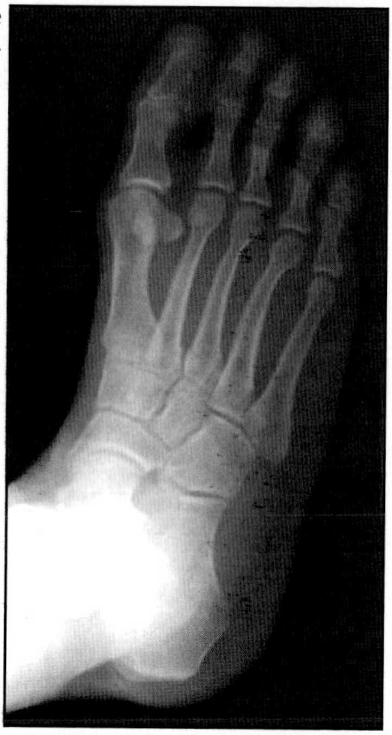

Figure 3-1B. Weight-bearing oblique view of the foot. Note rare sesamoids beneath metatarsal heads 2 and 5.

Oblique projection (Figure 3-1B) shows the following:

1. Relationships of lateral tarsometatarsal articulation: The medial edge of the fourth metatarsal shaft should align precisely with the medial edge of the cuboid.
2. One often has a particularly good view of the neck of the talus, the calcaneocuboid, and talonavicular joints on this view.

Lateral projection (Figure 3-1C) shows the following:

1. Arch height.
2. On a true lateral projection of the foot or ankle, the fibula should either completely be overlapped by the tibia or lie just posterior to it. One should not be able to see the entire width of the fibular shaft without any overlap. The ability to do so indicates a malpositioned limb or a lower extremity deformity.
3. Traction osteophytes can often be seen on the plantar and dorsal aspects of the calcaneal tuberosity, the latter of which may correlate with symptomatic insertional

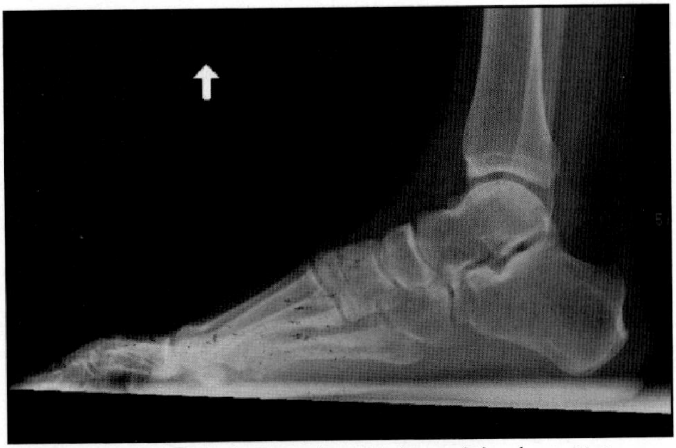

Figure 3-1C. Weight-bearing lateral view of the foot. Note rare sesamoids beneath metatarsal heads 2 and 5.

Achilles tendinopathy. While commonly thought to be the case, a plantar calcaneal spur is not associated with symptomatic plantar fasciitis.

4. Anterosuperior beaking of the anterior process of the calcaneus is suggestive of a calcaneonavicular coalition.
5. Dorsal osteophytes on the first metatarsal head are significant for degenerative changes at the first MTPJ.
6. The sesamoids should lie beneath the head of the first metatarsal but not the shaft; proximal migration suggests fracture or plantar plate injury.
7. Bohler's angle measures the degree of compression and deformity resulting from a calcaneus fracture. It is an angle formed by lines drawn from 1) the superior aspect of the anterior process of the calcaneus to the superior aspect of the posterior articular surface, and 2) from the superior aspect of the posterior articular surface to the superior aspect of the calcaneal tuberosity (normal 25 to 40 degrees).[2]
8. Crucial angle of Gissane provides a guide to the normal relationship between the anterior middle and posterior facets of the calcaneus, which can be disrupted in a calcaneus fracture. Formed by lines drawn along the thick sclerotic bone forming a "V" from the anterior process

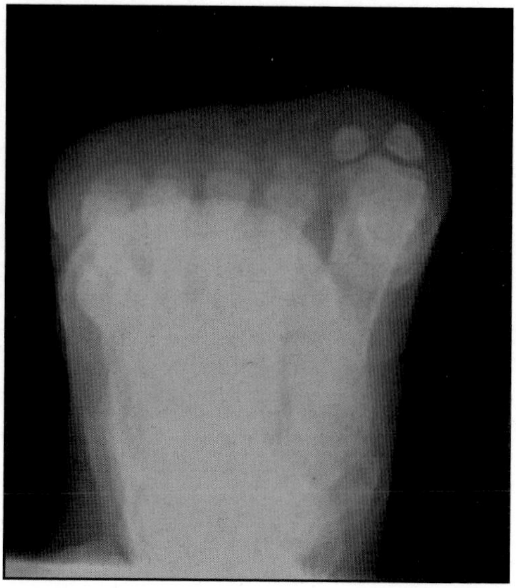

Figure 3-2. Sesamoid view of the foot.

of the calcaneus then along the posterior facet (normal 120 to 145 degrees).[2]

9. Meary's angle helps to determine degree of collapse or height of arch and is measured by the angle formed between the longitudinal axis of the talus and the longitudinal axis of the first metatarsal. These lines should be parallel. A positive angle (>0) indicates cavus, while a negative angle suggest a planus deformity.[2]

Special Views

Sesamoid view (Figure 3-2) is performed with the great toe dorsiflexed and beam directed to image the sesamoid-metatarsal articulation.

Canale view (Figure 3-3) visualizes the talar neck and is helpful for assessing reduction versus displacement of talar neck fractures.

Axial heel (Harris) view (Figure 3-4) visualizes the posterior facet of the subtalar joint as well as the middle facet/sustentaculum tali and any varus or valgus malalignment of the calcaneal tuberosity.

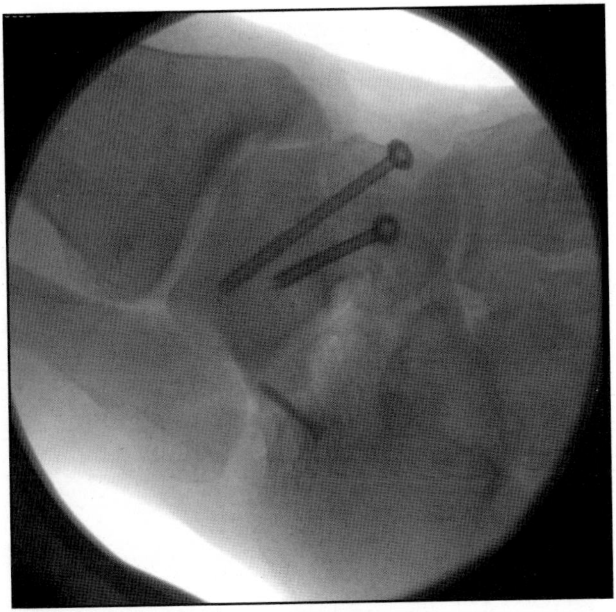

Figure 3-3. Canale view.

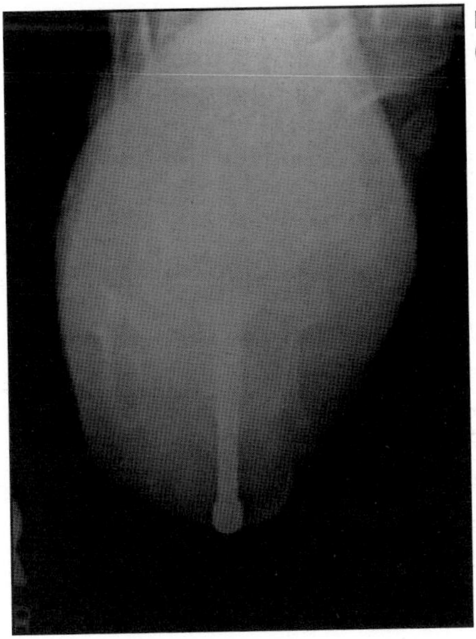

Figure 3-4. Axial heel (Harris) view.

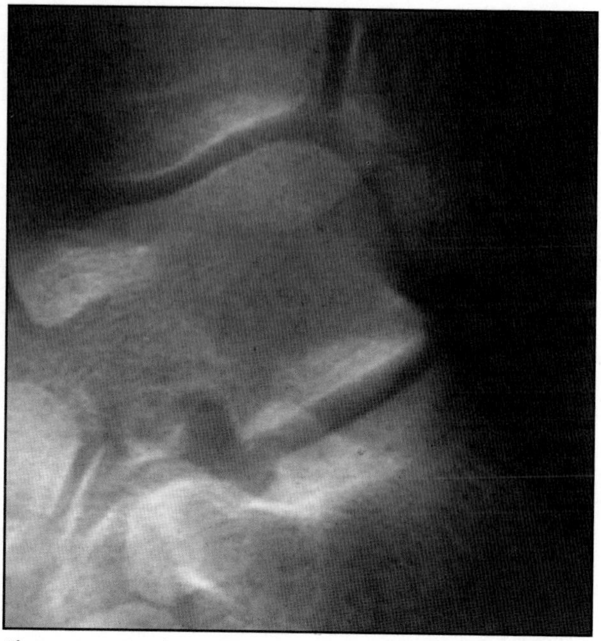

Figure 3-5. Broden's view

Broden's view (Figure 3-5) allows us to better image the posterior facet of the subtalar joint. This is often helpful using fluoroscopy during open reduction and internal fixation of calcaneus fractures involving displacement of the posterior facet.

Stress views (Figure 3-6) are often used to assess ligament stability and should be performed while wearing radioprotective gloves. Lateral ankle ligament instability and Lisfranc's disruptions are 2 entities whose diagnosis can be aided by stress radiographs.

Plain Radiography of the Ankle

Standard views of the ankle include AP, mortise, and lateral projections. These views are most useful in identifying pathology at the tibiotalar joint and checking the normal relationships between the tibia, talus, and fibula that may be altered as the result of trauma. Of particular importance is to make note of the fact that with the knees facing forward, the ankle joint

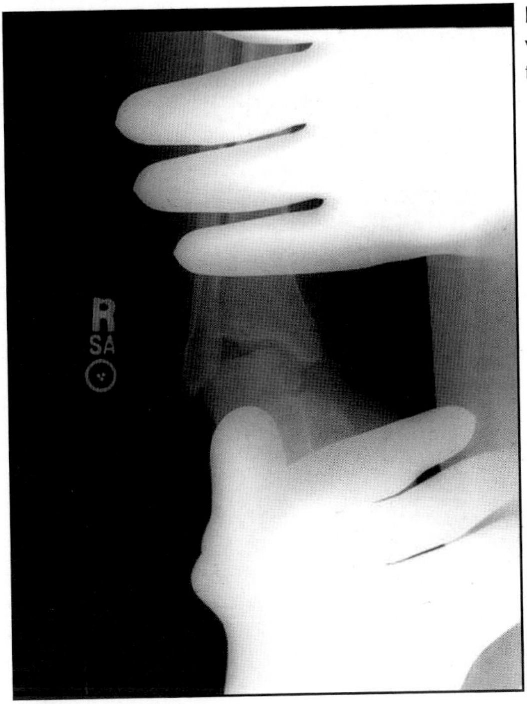

Figure 3-6. Stress view of the ankle—talar tilt view.

is slightly externally rotated and the fibula lies just posterior to the center of the tibia in the coronal plane. For this reason, an AP view of the ankle demonstrates considerable overlap of these 2 bones and only through internally rotating the limb can one see both the fibula and tibia in their entirety and their respective joint spaces (the mortise). As a lateral x-ray of the ankle often includes the foot, many of the aforementioned items seen on the lateral foot x-ray can similarly be seen on the lateral ankle projection.

AP projection (Figure 3-7A) shows the following:

1. Degenerative changes at the tibiotalar joint should be looked for here with attention to any malalignment.
2. Osteochondral lesions of the talus (OLTs) can be seen here.
3. The tibiofibular clear space is the space between the distal fibula and tibia and it should be less than 5 mm.
4. The tibia and fibula should overlap laterally at least 10 mm.

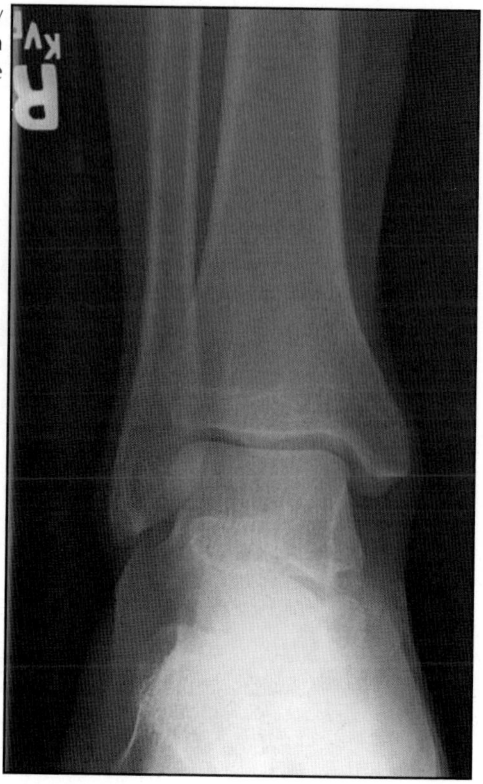

Figure 3-7A. AP view of the ankle. Note fifth metatarsal base fracture on lateral image.

Mortise view (20 degrees internally rotated ankle in neutral) (Figure 3-7B) shows the following:

1. The medial clear space is the space between the lateral surface of the medial malleolus and the medial surface of the talus. Normally the joint space between the tibia and talus, fibula and lateral talus, and medial malleolus and medial malleolus should be symmetric. The medial clear space indicates injury to the syndesmosis and should be within 2 mm of the remaining joint spaces referred to above and no more than 4 mm.

Lateral projection (Figure 3-7C) shows the following:

1. The posterior process of the talus may be seen as a long process from the talus or as a separate bone (os trigonum).

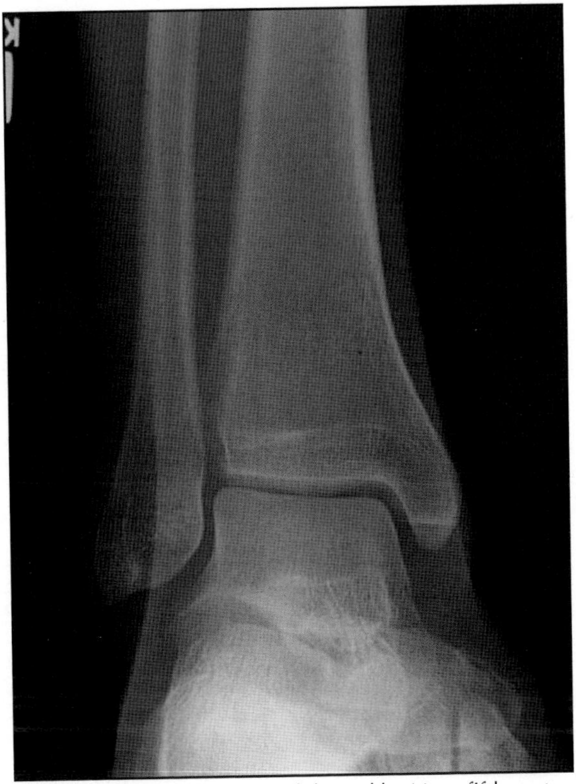

Figure 3-7B. Mortise view of the ankle. Note fifth metatarsal base fracture on lateral image.

2. Anterior osteophytes on the distal tibia suggest degenerative changes.
3. OLTs can also be viewed on the lateral projection.
4. Talonavicular arthritis and midfoot degenerative changes can be seen here.
5. The plantar aspect of a fifth metatarsal fracture can often be seen on this view.
6. NB: External rotation and anterior drawer stress views can be performed wearing lead gloves to aid in the diagnosis of ankle instability. Contralateral comparison films are particularly useful in assessing for generalized laxity in the setting of symptomatic instability.

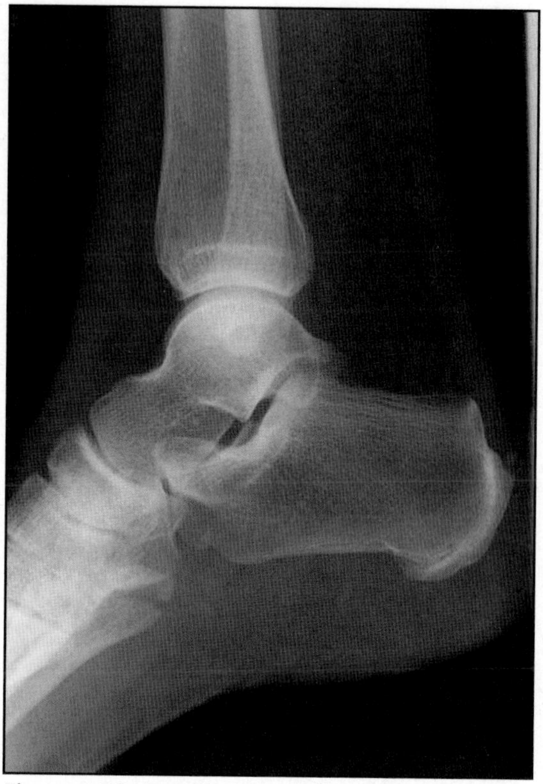

Figure 3-7C. Lateral view of the ankle. Note fifth metatarsal base fracture on lateral image.

Computed Tomography

Computed tomography (CT) of the foot and ankle is a non–weight-bearing modality that provides rapid imaging of very thin sections to help evaluate complex anatomy and pathology. This imaging modality is most useful in evaluating bone as opposed to soft tissue. CT is obtained through the use of a fan-shaped rotating x-ray beam that delivers radiation and obtains images in the axial plane only. The images can be obtained quickly with the use of newer machines that acquire images in a helical or spiral "scan." Pixels are displayed on a grayscale that is based on Hounsfield units (water being

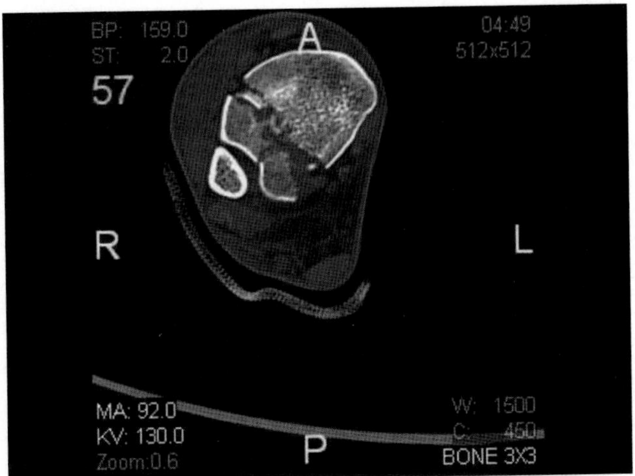

Figure 3-8A. CT ankle: Axial image of a distal tibia fracture.

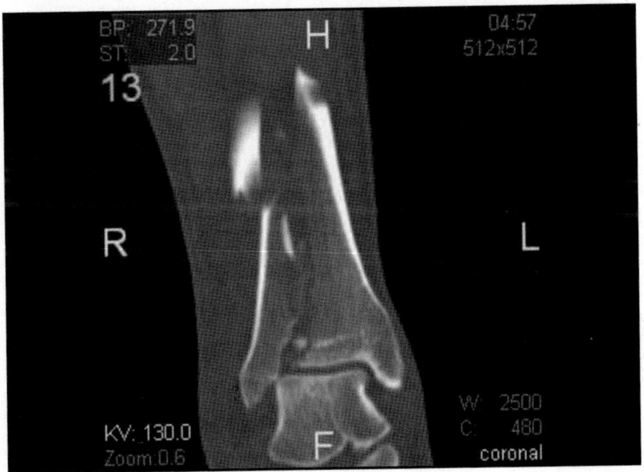

Figure 3-8B. CT ankle: Coronal image of a distal tibia fracture.

0, air being –1000, and bone having a value around +1000).[2] Through imaging software programs, reformatted coronal, sagittal, and 3-dimensional images can also be obtained. CT is particularly useful in preoperative planning because bony defects, complex relationships between structures, and the direction of fracture lines and planes can be more easily appreciated (Figure 3-8A to D).

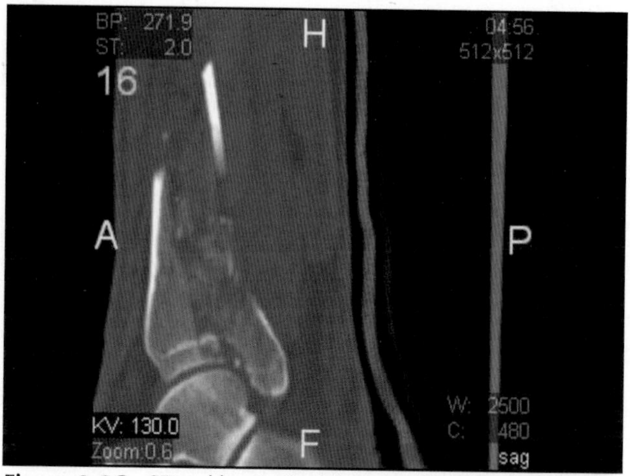

Figure 3-8C. CT ankle. Sagittal images of a distal tibia fracture.

Figure 3-8D. CT ankle. Preoperative plain film AP x-ray for comparison.

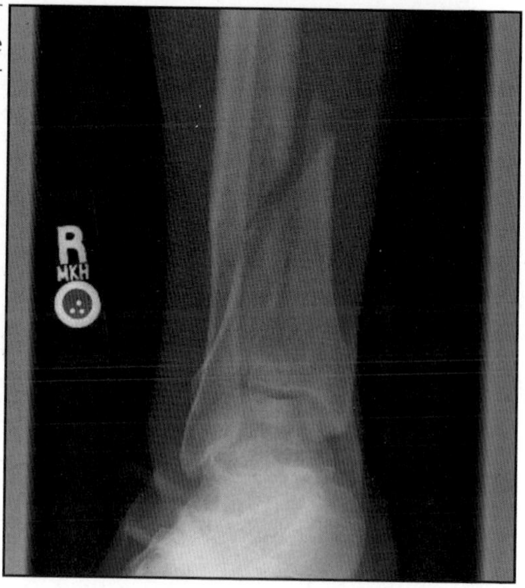

A note should be made on imaging for hindfoot trauma; calcaneus fracture classification, research, and treatment are commonly based on the alignment of the posterior facet of the subtalar joint. When a patient is lying on a CT gantry, however, there is considerable variability in the alignment of the posterior facet to the x-ray beam. For this reason, CT scans of the calcaneus following a fracture should specifically be obtained perpendicular to the posterior facet.

A few entities which CT is particularly useful in imaging include the following:

- Tarsal coalition (bony)
- Posterior malleolar fractures
- Bony loose bodies following reduction of a dislocated joint
- Calcaneus fractures
- Intra-articular distal tibia fractures
- Fractures of the talus
- Osteochondral lesions of the talus
- Navicular stress fractures
- Nonunions
- Bony tumors

Magnetic Resonance Imaging

Magnetic resonance imaging (MRI) is the most commonly used imaging modality for the evaluation of soft tissue pathology for the musculoskeletal system. Like CT scanning, MRI is a non–weight-bearing modality. Images are obtained using a large shielded magnet that aligns proton nuclei in a magnetic field. Once aligned, a radiofrequency is quickly delivered and displaces the protons that subsequently relax to their original positions. The time to relaxation is different for every tissue and is displayed on a grayscale. Images are acquired in the axial, coronal, and sagittal planes. Smaller extremities like the hand, elbow, foot, and ankle are often placed in a focusing "extremity coil" to further narrow the magnetic field (less scatter of the field) for more precise imaging.

An advantage of MRI is that one can obtain multiplanar images of soft tissues with exquisite detail without radiation exposure. Magnetic resonance arthrograms and angiograms can also be obtained. Disadvantages of MRI include poor bony detail compared to CT, patients must remain still during the study (failure to do so can lead to motion artifacts), some

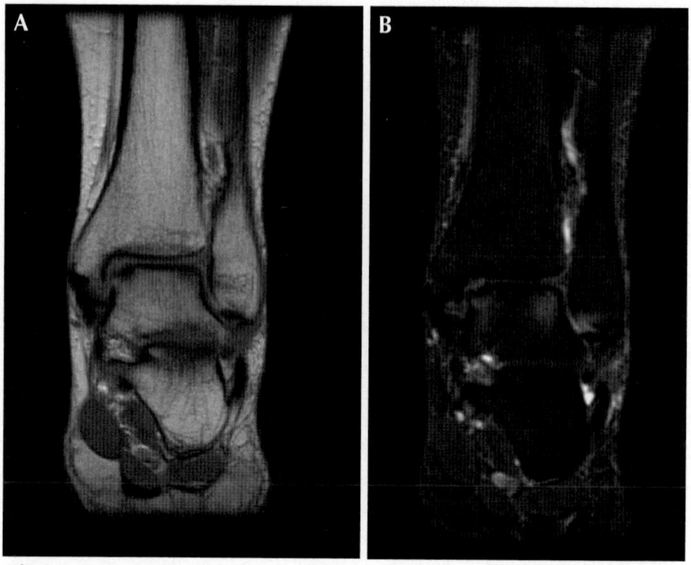

Figure 3-9. MRI ankle T1 weighted coronal view (A) reveals large medial and smaller lateral osteochondral lesions of the talus with corresponding edema seen on T2 weighted image (B).

patients become claustrophobic during the study, and lastly, retained ferrous-based metal implants greatly obscure the images. Patients with loose metal bodies near vital structures, older defibrillators, and vascular clips in the brain are often contraindicated to undergo MRI.

A few entities which MRI is particularly useful in imaging include the following:

- Tarsal coalition (fibrous)
- Osteochondral lesions of the talus (Figure 3-9)
- Bony and soft tissue tumors of the foot and ankle
- Tendon tears
- Tendinopathy
- Stress reactions
- Bone bruises
- Navicular stress fractures
- Ligament tears
- Differentiating sesamoid and plantar plate complex pathology

Ultrasonography

Musculoskeletal ultrasound has been used for decades in many centers but has recently seen a resurgence in its use, likely due to its advantages of being inexpensive, readily available in most radiology departments, and its lack of ionizing radiation exposure. It is particularly suited for soft tissue imaging.

Ultrasound is not able to visualize bony pathology effectively and cannot be used through a cast. The major disadvantage of this imaging modality is that the results are largely operator dependant and considerable variability can be seen in the quality and interpretation of images. For this reason, many remain cautious about musculoskeletal ultrasound's ability to accurately diagnose acute and chronic pathology.

Musculoskeletal ultrasound of the foot and ankle can be particularly helpful in diagnosing the following:

- Tendon degeneration
- Tendon rupture
- Peritendinitis
- Lateral ankle ligament tears
- Guided aspirations or biopsies
- Subtalar instability
- Wooden foreign bodies

Nuclear Medicine

Nuclear medicine uses intravenously administered radioactive isotope tracers and gamma cameras to acquire images at various time intervals to depict the flow and metabolism of various compounds in the body. Two of the most commonly used modalities in orthopedic surgery are 3-phase bone scan and tagged white blood cell (WBC) scan.

Bone scans use technetium 99m methylene diphosphonate (99mTc MDP) as a tracer. This tracer binds to hydroxyapetite crystals in forming bone, thus it is useful in imaging conditions in which bone is being turned over. Bone tumors, infections, and occult fractures have long been imaged using bone scans. Typically, images are assessed in 3 phases. The first

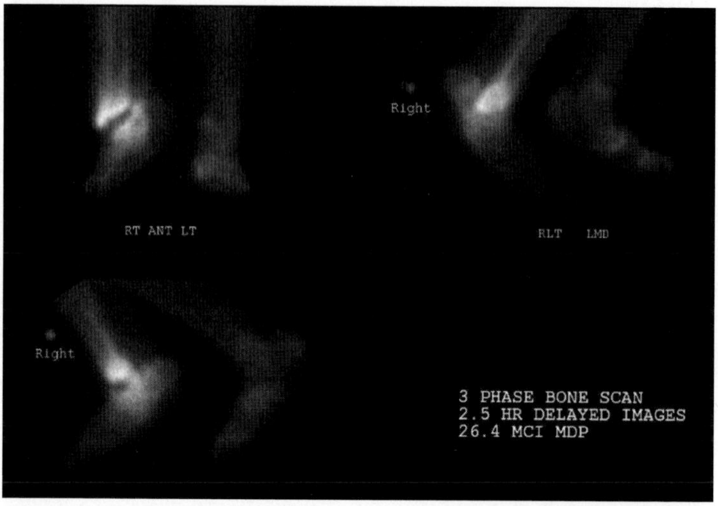

Figure 3-10. Three-phase bone scan of the lower extremity. This is a case of osteomyelitis of the ankle.

phase following injection is the blood flow phase (up to 60 seconds following injection). The second phase or blood pool is at 5 minutes and the third phase, also known as the bone turnover phase, is typically acquired at 4 hours postinjection.[2]

WBC scans involve labeling a patient's sampled WBCs usually with indium. The tagged cells are then injected back into the patient and imaged at around 24 hours to see where those leukocytes have congregated. Since WBCs are those that predominate in a response to an infection (ie, osteomyelitis), tagged WBC scans are often used to diagnose bone infections. Typically indium scans are compared to bone scans for the same patient to differentiate infection from other bony pathology. This comparison is particularly helpful in separating those with positive bone scans seen in diabetic Charcot neuropathy from those who have osteomyelitis.

Nuclear imaging of the foot and ankle can be particularly helpful in diagnosing the following:

- Metastatic tumor
- Infection (Figure 3-10)
- Stress reaction/early stress fracture
- Complex regional pain syndrome

Conclusion

Secondary only to our history taking and physical examination, musculoskeletal imaging allows us to accurately and quickly render diagnoses and treatment in a way no other aspect of medicine has affected orthopedic surgery. Being able to deliver a high standard of care is predicated on a thorough understanding of plain radiography, CT, MRI, ultrasound, and nuclear medicine. Hopefully, this chapter has served as an introduction to this topic and we recommend further study with the aid of formal radiology and orthopedic texts.

References

1. Stiell IG, Greenberg GH, McKnight RD, Nair RC, McDowell I, Worthington JR. A study to develop clinical decision rules for the use of radiography in acute ankle injuries. *Ann Emerg Med.* 1992;21(4):384-390.
2. Coughlin M, Mann R, Saltzman C. Imaging of the foot and ankle. In: *Surgery of the Foot and Ankle* 8th ed. Philadelphia, PA: Elsevier; 2007:71-131.

Suggested Readings

Erkonen WE, Smith WL. *Radiology 101: The Basics and Fundamentals of Imaging.* Philadelphia, PA: Lippincott Williams & Wilkins; 2009.

Pope T, Morrison WB, Bloom HL, Wilson DJ. *Imaging of the Musculoskeletal System: Expert Radiology Series.* St. Louis, MO: WB Saunders; 2008.

III

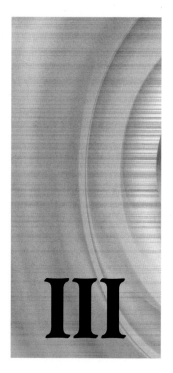

Common Conditions of the Foot and Ankle

4

Ankle Instability

Seth R. Queler, MD

Introduction

Chronic ankle instability is defined as recurrent *giving way* of the ankle and manifests after multiple ankle sprains, more commonly if they are left untreated. Ankle sprains are the most common injuries in athletes.[1] It is estimated that in the United States, over 23 000 ankle sprains occur every day.[2] While ankle sprains are extremely common, most patients who experience ankle sprains do not develop chronic ankle instability. Ankle instability can be classified as either lateral or medial. The lateral ligament complex includes the anterior talofibular ligament (ATFL), calcaneofibular ligament (CFL), and posterior talofibular ligament (PTFL), while the medial

Hurwitz SR, Parekh SG. *Musculoskeletal Examination of the Foot and Ankle: Making the Complex Simple* (pp. 59-77). © 2012 SLACK Incorporated.

ligament complex includes the deltoid ligament and the spring (calcaneonavicular) ligament. Lateral ankle sprains, which are far more common than the medial type, occur due to an inversion ankle injury in a plantarflexed foot. In the meantime, injury to the medial ligament complex is secondary to eversion ankle injury.

Ankle instability can also be classified as either mechanical or functional. Mechanical ankle instability is defined as abnormal laxity of ankle ligaments found on physical exam. Functional ankle instability refers to the subjective complaint of the ankle giving way and has been attributed to neuromuscular and proprioceptive deficits.[3] The presenting patient can have either mechanical or functional instability or both. Therefore, a patient with functional ankle instability and no mechanical instability will complain of recurrent sprains without any physical sign of laxity on exam (Table 4-1).

History

Patients with ankle instability present to the clinician with a history of multiple ankle sprains. If there has been previous injury, the clinician should ascertain what type of treatment has been provided to the patient in the past. Does the patient wear a brace? Has the patient had any rehabilitation or previous ankle surgery? If the patient has had physical therapy in the past, it is important to determine what types of exercises were performed and for how long they were performed. While lateral ankle instability is much more common, the clinician should ask the patient the direction of his or her instability. Therefore, the mechanism of injury is extremely important when obtaining a history. Patients with lateral ankle instability give a history of an inversion injury in a plantarflexed foot. A history of an eversion injury is typical in patients with medial ankle instability. The patient with an acute injury may report a history of previous sprains. Since patients with acute injuries may not volunteer this information, it is crucial that the clinician carefully question the patient about this part of his or her history. Patients often report a sense of "looseness," "weakness," or "giving way" and a fear of another sprain or episode. They complain of difficulty with walking on uneven terrain.

Table 4-1

Helpful Hints

Types of Instability

Direction	Mechanism of Injury	Injured Ligament(s)
Medial	Eversion	Deltoid ligaments +/– spring ligament
Lateral	Plantar flexion-inversion	ATFL +/– CFL

Type	History	Physical Exam
Functional	Patient complains of giving way or instability	Negative instability on exam (anterior drawer or talar tilt)
Mechanical	History of ankle injury	Positive instability on exam (anterior drawer or talar tilt)

Imaging

Image	Pertinent Views	Findings
Foot series radiographs	Anteroposterior (AP), oblique, lateral	Rule out associated injuries (Lisfranc's injury, base of fifth metatarsal fracture, cuboid fracture, anterior process calcaneus fracture)
Ankle series radiographs	AP, mortise, lateral	Rule out associated injuries (osteochondral lesion of talus fracture, Shepherd's fracture, syndesmotic injury, lateral process talus fracture)
Stress radiograph	Anterior drawer, talar tilt	Anterior drawer <10 mm (<3 mm side-to-side difference) Talar tilt <10 degrees (<5 degrees side-to-side difference)
MRI/CT	Axial, coronal, sagittal	Rule out associated injuries (those noted above, tendon pathology, occult fractures)

Another common symptom is pain, which may or may not be related to a recent sprain. When evaluating the patient with ankle instability, it is critical to determine whether the patient was able to bear weight after the injury or injuries. If pain is present, an associated injury should be considered. Other injuries that are often missed but may be present include Lisfranc's injury, osteochondral lesion of the talus, peroneal tendon tear or dislocation, syndesmotic injury, peripheral nerve injury, or fracture of the base of the fifth metatarsal, anterior process of the calcaneus, lateral process of the talus, cuboid, Stieda's process (Shepherd's fracture), or navicular. Associated injuries are not uncommon in patients with chronic lateral ankle instability. The most common associated ankle injuries are peroneal tenosynovitis, anterolateral ankle impingement, and ankle synovitis.[4] For this reason, it is vital that the clinician asks the patient the exact location of his or her pain. Numbness or paresthesias on the dorsum of the foot may be related to previous traction injuries to the superficial peroneal nerve status postinversion injuries. Another complaint may be swelling. In addition, an important question to ask prior to examination is if the patient injured the opposite side.

The past medical history, family history, and social history of the patient with ankle instability should not be overlooked by the clinician. The examiner should also determine if the patient has a history of any previous dislocations such as patellar or shoulder dislocations. Previous dislocation may indicate that the patient has generalized ligamentous laxity, and this is important when considering how to tailor a treatment plan for the patient. Is there a family history of Charcot-Marie-Tooth or collagen disease that may put the patient at risk for ankle instability? What is the patient's occupation? What is the patient's activity level in sports?

EXAMINATION

The physical examination of the patient with ankle instability should include examination of the lower extremity from just below the knee down to the foot (Table 4-2). A complete examination should include inspection, palpation, range of motion, strength testing, and provocative maneuvers of both lower

Table 4-2

METHODS FOR EXAMINING THE UNSTABLE ANKLE

Examination	*Technique*	*Illustration*	*Grading/Characteristics*	*Significance*
Inspection	Examine for swelling	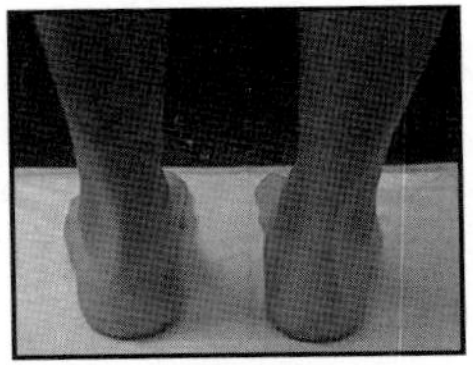		
	Examine gait	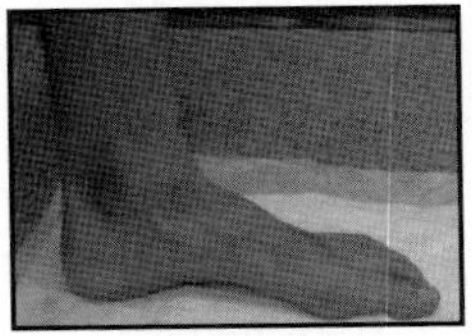	Hindfoot varus Pes cavus	Places lateral ligaments and tendons at risk for injury
	Examine for malalignment	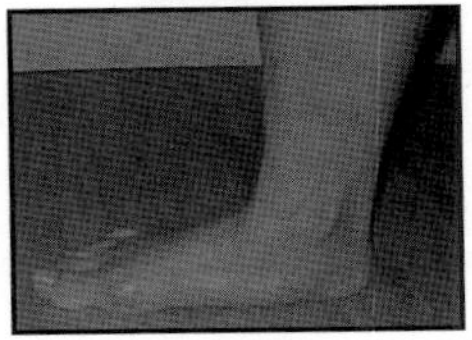	Hindfoot valgus Pes planus	Places medial ligaments and tendons at risk for injury

(continued)

Table 4-2 (continued)

Methods for Examining the Unstable Ankle

Examination	*Technique*	*Illustration*	*Grading/Characteristics*	*Significance*
Inspection	Examine for skin, hair pattern, nails			
	Examine for atrophy		Peroneal wasting	Charcot-Marie-Tooth disease
Range of motion	Examine active and passive ankle range of motion			Loss of active motion may be related to pain
				Loss of passive motion may be due to contracture
	Dorsiflexion			
	Plantar flexion			
	Subtalar motion			
	Inversion			
	Eversion			
Palpation	Examine leg, ankle and foot ATFL CFL Peroneal tendons		Positive: tenderness	Rule out associated injury

(continued)

Table 4-2 (continued)

METHODS FOR EXAMINING THE UNSTABLE ANKLE

Examination	*Technique*	*Illustration*	*Grading/Characteristics*	*Significance*
Palpation (continued)	Deltoid ligament Fibula—entire length Medial malleolus Talus Posterior tibial tendon Base of fifth metatarsal Lisfranc's joint AITFL Achilles		Positive: tenderness	Rule out associated injury
Strength testing	Examine strength of dorsiflexion (external rotation) and plantar flexion (inversion)	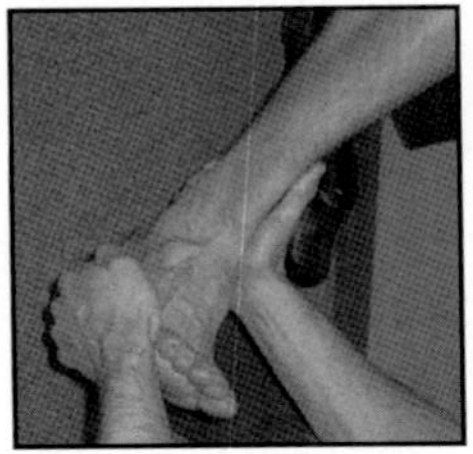	Grade 5 = Full strength against resistance Grade 4 = Less than full strength against resistance Grade 3 = Movement against gravity Grade 2 = Movement with gravity Grade 1 = Visible muscle contraction Grade 0 = No movement	Peroneal weakness indicates peroneal dysfunction or under-rehabilitated lateral ankle sprain Posterior tibial tendon strength

(continued)

Table 4-2 (continued)

Methods for Examining the Unstable Ankle

Provocative Tests

Examination	Technique	Illustration	Grading/Characteristics	Significance
Anterior drawer	With ankle in 10 to 15 degrees plantar flexion ankle translated anteriorly under tibia	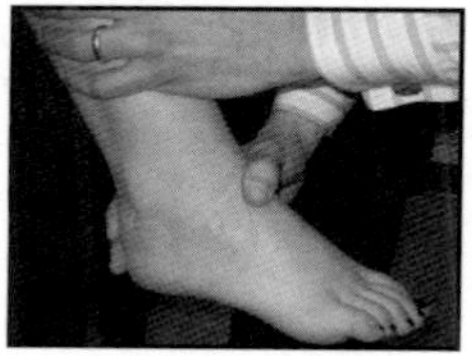		ATFL tear
	With ankle in neutral dorsiflexion-plantar flexion ankle translated anteriorly under tibia	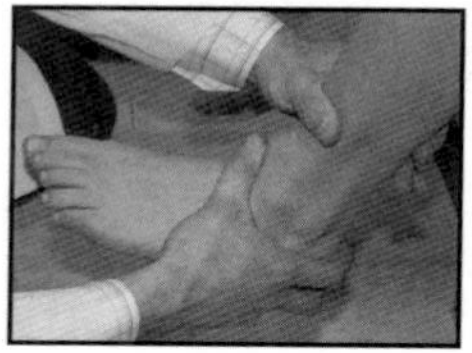		CFL tear
Sulcus sign			Noted anterior to fibula	Complete tear of the ATFL
Talar tilt	Inversion stress to the heel	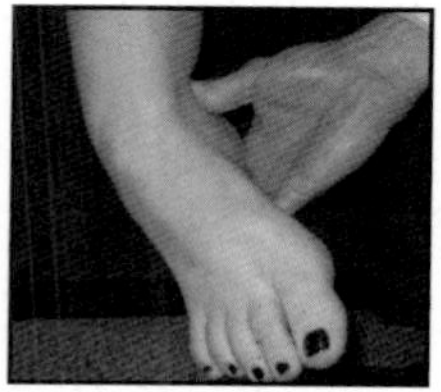		ATFL and CFL tear

(continued)

Table 4-2 (continued)

Methods for Examining the Unstable Ankle

Provocative Tests

Examination	Technique	Illustration	Grading/Characteristics	Significance
Eversion stress test	Eversion stress to the heel			Deltoid ligament tear
Squeeze test	Squeeze tibia and fibular together at midcalf	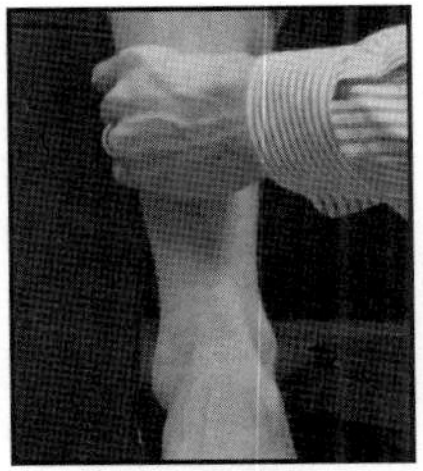	Positive: pain at ankle	Syndesmotic injury
External rotation test	Passive dorsiflexion-external rotation of foot	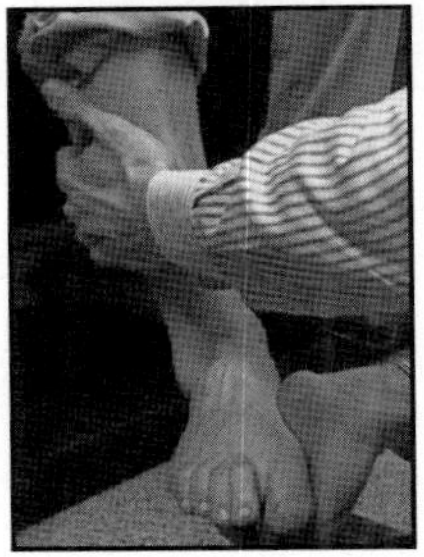	Positive: pain	Syndesmotic injury

(continued)

Table 4-2 (continued)

Methods for Examining the Unstable Ankle

Provocative Tests

Examination	Technique	Illustration	Grading/Characteristics	Significance
Thompson test	Squeeze calf for passive plantar flexion of the foot	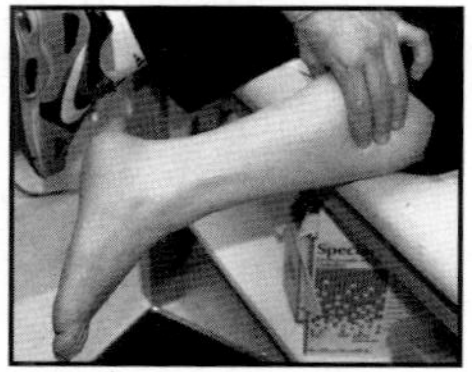	Positive: foot does not plantarflex	Achilles rupture
Ligamentous laxity	Tests: thumb to forearm; passive MCP extension of small finger >90 degrees; elbow hyperextension; knee hyperextension; sulcus sign; palms flat to floor		Beighton Ligamentous Laxity Scale (score 0 to 3 = tight, 4 to 6 = hypermobile; 7 to 9 = excessive hypermobility)[5]	Positive finding may predispose to instability and failure of ligament repair
Coleman block test	Place medial forefoot on block in a patient with hindfoot varus	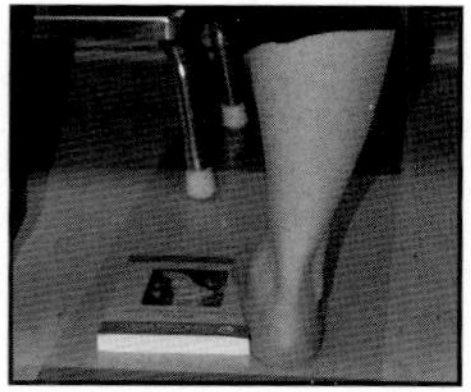	Hindfoot alignment corrects Hindfoot alignment does not correct	Flexible hindfoot varus Rigid hindfoot varus

extremities in order to compare the 2 sides for any side-to-side differences. Generalized ligamentous laxity may predispose the patient to ankle instability and should be determined on physical examination using the Beighton Ligamentous Laxity Scale.[5] In addition, the patient's gait should be observed. Part of the exam includes inspection of the patient's shoes and any bracing that is utilized by the patient. The shoes can specifically be examined for any particular wear patterns that could indicate hindfoot misalignment. The examination should also include determination of the dorsalis pedis and posterior tibial pulses and a complete sensory examination.

Inspection of the patient in both sitting and standing positions is an important part of the physical examination (Table 4-3). The patient should be examined with the legs hanging off the side of the examination table with the knees flexed 90 degrees. The examiner should specifically observe any misalignment of the foot and ankle. Hindfoot varus or pes cavus deformity can predispose the patient to lateral ligament injury and subsequent instability. If pes cavus is present, a Coleman block test should be performed. Planovalgus, pes planus deformity, and "too many toes" sign can predispose the patient to injury to the medial ankle structures. In addition, the examiner should note the presence of any swelling in the foot or ankle and whether this swelling is focal or diffuse. If there is swelling, it should be determined if this is associated with an ankle effusion, which may indicate intra-articular pathology such as osteochondral lesion of the talus. Inspection of the legs, ankles, and feet should also include examination of the skin and hair pattern, rashes, ulceration, calluses, and nails. The presence of atrophy is extremely important. Patients with Charcot-Marie-Tooth disease may have atrophy at the level of the peroneal muscles. Range of motion of the ankle, subtalar joint, and transverse tarsal joints should be evaluated while noting any crepitation or pain. Palpation should also include determination for any focal tenderness. This is critical in determining any associated injury. Specifically palpate all bony prominences, joints, ligaments, muscles, and tendons. The fibula should be palpated along its entire length to rule out any fracture. The ATFL, CFL, deltoid ligament, and anterior inferior tib-fib ligament (AITFL) should be palpated. The peroneal, Achilles, and posterior tibial tendons should also be palpated to rule out tendon tear or rupture or peroneal tendon subluxation/dislocation. Strength testing should include plantar flexion, dorsiflexion, and plantar flexion-inversion testing. In particular, dorsiflexion-eversion strength is particularly important in determining peroneal strength, which should be 5/5 in a normal exam. Any peroneal strength deficit may indicate peroneal dysfunction or an under-rehabilitated ankle, which has been shown to contribute to lateral ankle instability.[6]

Provocative maneuvers are an important part of the physical exam. Anterior drawer and talar tilt tests should be performed with the legs hanging off the side of the examination table with the knees bent at 90 degrees. The anterior drawer test should be performed with the ankle in slight plantar flexion to test the ATFL and with the ankle in neutral to test the CFL. The ankle should be allowed to rotate medially to relax the deltoid while the foot is translated anteriorly with the tibia stabilized with the opposite hand. A sulcus sign can be present in patients with a complete tear of the ATFL. A positive talar tilt test is an indication of injury to both ATFL and CFL, but this test can be unreliable due to variations in subtalar motion.[7,8] The deltoid ligament may be tested through eversion stress testing. A squeeze test and an external rotation test should be performed to rule out syndesmotic injury. A Thompson test should be performed in the presence of acute injury to rule out an Achilles tendon rupture. A positive Tinel's sign can indicate peripheral nerve injury. Not uncommonly, lateral ankle sprains may also include traction injury to the superficial peroneal nerve, which can lead to lateral ankle pain or foot numbness.

Pathoanatomy

Ankle sprains are graded 1, 2, or 3. A grade 1 ankle sprain is a stretch injury while grade 2 and 3 sprains are partial and complete ligament tear injuries, respectively. Misalignment of the lower extremity predisposes the patient to ankle instability. A patient with cavovarus deformity places the lateral ankle ligaments at risk for injury. In addition, patients with generalized ligamentous laxity are predisposed to ankle instability.

The lateral ligament complex includes the ATFL, CFL, and PTFL while the medial ligament complex includes the deltoid ligament and the spring ligament complex. While the ATFL crosses only the ankle joint, the CFL traverses both the ankle and the subtalar joints. The most common ligament injury in a lateral ankle sprain is to the ATFL since the most common ankle sprain occurs with the ankle in plantar flexion and inversion, placing maximal stretch on the ATFL. In addition, the ATFL is weaker than the CFL, which is tight with the ankle in neutral. Also very common is a combination injury of ATFL and CFL which occurs in more severe sprains. Rarely, the PTFL is injured in lateral ankle sprains. Lateral ligament injuries are more commonly midsubstance sprains, but they can result in avulsion injuries.[9] Incompetence of the ATFL correlates with a positive anterior drawer on exam. A positive talar tilt test is indicative of injury to both the ATFL and the CFL.[3,10] Medial ankle instability has been divided into 3 types. A type I lesion includes a proximal deltoid tear or avulsion, a type II lesion includes an intermediate deltoid tear, and a type III lesion includes a distal deltoid tear or avulsion and a spring ligament tear.[11]

The lateral ankle ligaments and the bony anatomy act as static stabilizers of the ankle and hindfoot. Injury to the ligaments leads to mechanical ankle instability. The peroneal muscle-tendon units act as dynamic stabilizers. Lateral ankle instability is caused by deficits in ligamentous integrity, muscle strength, and proprioception. Patients with chronic ankle instability are known to have weakness, although this is not always present. Proprioception and neuromuscular deficits are known to contribute to functional ankle instability.[3] Patients often have a combination of both mechanical and functional ankle instability. These underlying deficits help plan and direct treatment for instability.

IMAGING

A weight-bearing ankle series should include AP, lateral, and mortise x-rays. The mortise view is a 20-degree internal rotation view of the ankle. If the patient is noted to have proximal fibular tenderness, then an AP and lateral tib-fib series

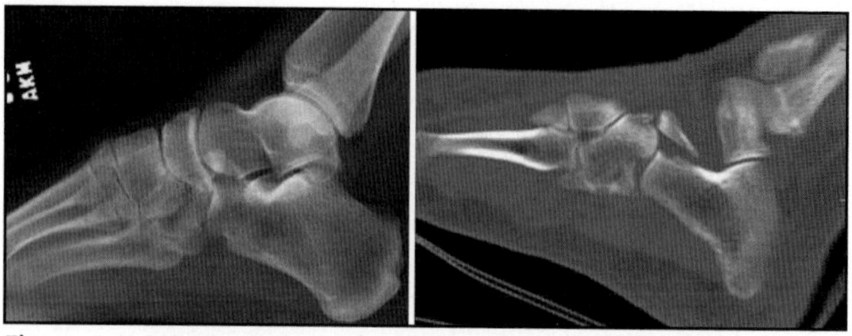

Figure 4-1. Anterior process of calcaneus and cuboid fractures.

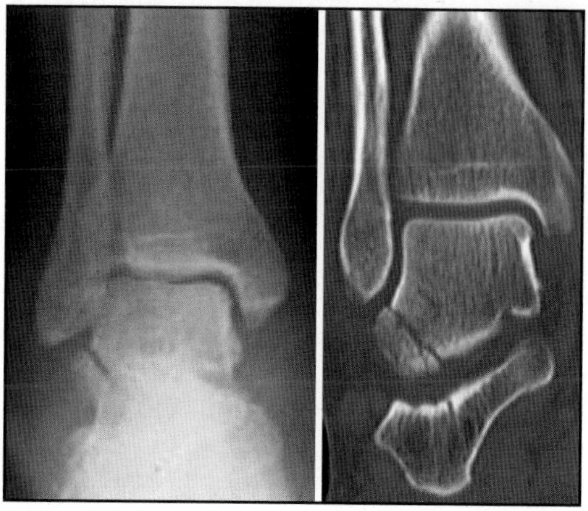

Figure 4-2. Lateral process talus fracture.

should also be obtained. Weight-bearing views allow accurate evaluation of ankle and subtalar joint alignment while non–weight-bearing x-rays can lead to misleading findings. Any varus or valgus ankle alignment should be noted. The syndesmosis should be inspected for any widening. The radiographs should be evaluated for any associated fractures of the foot and ankle such as lateral process fractures or osteochondral lesions of the talus, anterior process of the calcaneus fracture, or cuboid fractures (Figure 4-1). Tenderness at the level of the ATFL and the lateral process of the talus may be difficult to distinguish. Therefore, it is important to specifically rule out a lateral process of the talus fracture on radiograph for patients with tenderness in this region to distinguish ATFL injury and lateral process of the talus fracture (Figure 4-2). The x-rays

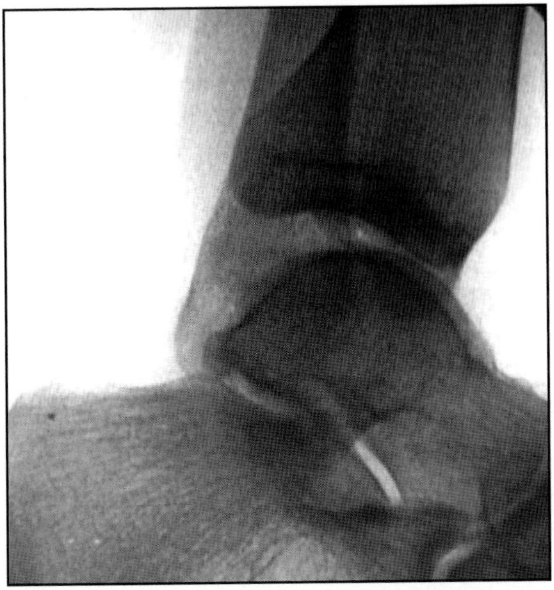

Figure 4-3. Anterior drawer stress test radiograph.

should also be examined for any degenerative changes including osteophyte formation and joint congruency. Anterior bony impingement can be identified and is typically observed with distal tibial osteophytes in patients with anterior ankle pain.

Anterior drawer and talar tilt stress views are somewhat controversial but can radiographically demonstrate ankle instability (Figure 4-3). Unfortunately, variability in stress views makes interpretation and standard measurements difficult. Meta-analysis has determined that stress radiography is too variable to reliably evaluate ankle instability.[12] However, stress views can be helpful to confirm the diagnosis, and comparison views may help to establish side-to-side differences. No standard measurements are available and recommendations vary. The anterior drawer should measure less than 10 mm absolute value or less than 3 mm difference when compared to the opposite side. The talar tilt should have an absolute value of less than 10 or 5 degrees when compared to the opposite side.[4]

Advanced imaging, such as magnetic resonance imaging (MRI) and computed tomography (CT), can be helpful when evaluating associated injuries that can occur in concordance with chronic ankle instability. Fractures, osteochondral injuries, and tendon pathology can be evaluated in detail with advanced imaging studies that are often present in the face of ankle instability. These studies and evaluation of concomitant injuries can help preoperatively plan and direct future treatment options.

Treatment

Less than 10% of patients that sustain an ankle sprain require future surgical repair or reconstruction of ankle ligaments.[13,14] Patients who suffer an acute ankle sprain should be treated initially with rest, ice, compression, elevation, and bracing for temporary mechanical stabilization. Bracing can come in the form of strapping, lace-up bracing, air stirrup bracing, or casting, depending of the severity of the injury and the patient's ability to bear weight. These devices provide sensory feedback that can improve proprioception. They also help add mechanical support to the unstable ankle but can sometimes be cumbersome.[15] In addition, both acute and chronic ankle instability should be treated with a formal rehabilitation program, often for 2 to 3 months, that is directed by the physician and overseen by the physical therapist. This program should begin once the patient's initial swelling and pain have subsided. The hallmarks of the physical therapy program for lateral ankle instability include peroneal muscle strengthening and proprioceptive training. Other modalities include range of motion and Achilles stretching, which should begin within 2 to 3 days after an acute sprain to prevent stiffness. Patients should perform a daily home exercise program both during and after completion of the formal rehabilitation program with the physical therapist. While both mechanical and functional ankle instability benefit from a structured physical therapy program, patients with functional instability are more likely to benefit.

If conservative management fails to improve lateral chronic mechanical ankle instability, then surgical intervention should be considered. Surgical stabilizing procedures are numerous and can be divided in 2 categories: anatomic repair with or without augmentation and ligament reconstruction utilizing tenodesis. Ligament reconstruction can be either anatomic or nonanatomic and utilizes either a local or distant autograft tendon or an allograft tendon. Anatomic repair of the ATFL +/– CFL was first described by Brostrom[16] in 1966. Gould later modified this procedure by augmenting the ligament repair by mobilizing the inferior extensor retinaculum of the ankle, a structure that crosses both the ankle and subtalar joints, and attaching it to the distal fibula.[17] One advantage of the modified Brostrom procedure, which has a success rate of approximately 90%, is restoration of the normal anatomy while preserving ankle and subtalar joint motion.[4,14] Due to the reliance on poor tissue, the modified Brostrom procedure has been less successful in patients with generalized ligament laxity.

There are numerous nonanatomic ligament reconstruction procedures that use tenodesis to provide stability to the unstable ankle. These procedures, which include Evans, Chrisman-Snook, and Watson-Jones, have shown short-term success, but long-term consequences include ankle arthritis.[18] In addition, these procedures can restrict normal subtalar motion[17,19] and often sacrifice part of or an entire peroneal tendon as autograft. More recently, anatomic reconstruction of the lateral ligaments with a free tendon graft has become a more popular surgical solution for lateral ankle instability. This includes the use of the tendon graft through bone tunnels in the talus, fibula, and calcaneus at the level of the origins and insertions of the ATFL and CFL. Advantages include preservation of the normal anatomy and avoiding the use of the peroneal tendons.[20] Indications for anatomic ankle ligament reconstruction include lateral ankle instability in patients with generalized ligamentous laxity or in patients with previously failed modified Brostrom procedure.

Other procedures should be considered for patients with ankle instability. Those patients with intra-articular ankle pathology should undergo ankle arthroscopy. A lateral slide calcaneal osteotomy should be performed for patients with underlying calcaneus varus deformity. Failure to correct such deformity will place the patient at a very high risk for failure of any ligament procedure.[20] In the meantime, medial ankle instability, which is less common, can be addressed by surgical reconstruction of the medial ligaments.[11]

Conclusion

Ankle sprains are very common injuries but associated injuries are often missed and should be ruled out in patients with ankle injuries. While lateral ankle instability is more common, medial ankle instability should not be overlooked. A thorough history and physical exam are critical in diagnosis and help dictate the optimal treatment plan. A physical therapy program should be used as the first line of treatment of both ankle sprains and chronic ankle instability. The current surgical treatment options include a modified Brostrom or lateral ligament repair with augmentation with the extensor retinaculum or ligament reconstruction with tenodesis. A free tendon autograft or allograft with anatomic reconstruction of the ankle ligaments has become the procedure of choice for patients who have lateral chronic ankle instability and generalized ligamentous laxity or have failed a modified Brostrom procedure.

References

1. Garrick JG. The frequency of injury mechanism of injury and epidemiology of ankle sprains. *Am J Sports Med.* 1977; 5(6):241-242.
2. Kannus P, Renström P. Treatment for acute tears of the lateral ligaments of the ankle: operation, cast, or early controlled mobilization. *J Bone Joint Surg Am.* 1991;73(2):305-312.
3. Hertel J. Functional instability following lateral ankle sprain. *Sports Med.* 2000;29(5):361-371.
4. DiGiovanni BF, Fraga CJ, Cohen BE, Shereff MJ. Associated injuries found in chronic lateral ankle instability. *Foot Ankle Int.* 2000;21(10):809-815.
5. Beighton PH, Horan FT. Dominant inheritance in familial generalised articular hypermobility. *J Bone Joint Surg Br.* 1970;52(1):145-147.
6. Wilkerson GB, Pinerola J, Caturano RW. Invertor vs. evertor peak torque and power deficiencies associated with lateral ankle ligament injury. *J Orthop Sports Phys Ther.* 1997;26(2):78-86.
7. Laurin CA, Ouellet R, St-Jacques R. Talar and subtalar tilt: an experimental investigation. *Can J Surg.* 1968;11(3):270-279.
8. Espinosa N, Smerek J, Kadakia AR, Myerson MS. Operative management of ankle instability: Reconstruction with open and percutaneous methods. *Foot Ankle Clin.* 2006;11(3):547-565.
9. Coughlin MJ, Mann RA, Saltzman CL. *Surgery of the Foot and Ankle.* 8th ed., Philadelphia, PA: Mosby Elsevier; 2007:1454.

10. Rasmussen O, Tovborg-Jensen I. Mobility of the ankle joint: recording and rotatory movements in the talocrural joint in vitro with and without the lateral collateral ligaments of the ankle. *Acta Orthop Scand.* 1982;53(1):155-160.
11. Hintermann B. Medial ankle instability. *Foot Ankle Clin.* 2003;8(4):723-738.
12. Frost SCL, Amendola A. Is stress radiography necessary in the diagnosis of acute or chronic ankle instability? *Clin J Sport Med.* 1999;9(1):40-45.
13. Karlsson J, Bergsten T, Lansinger O, Peterson, L. Reconstruction of the lateral ligaments of the ankle for chronic lateral instability. *J Bone Joint Surg Am.* 1988;70(4):581-588.
14. Krips R, de Vries J, van Dijk CN. Ankle instability. *Foot Ankle Clin.* 2006;11(2):311-329, vi.
15. Mattacola CG, Dwyer MK. Rehabilitation of the ankle after acute sprain or chronic instability. *J Athl Train.* 2002;37(4):413-429.
16. Broström L. Sprained ankles. 3. Clinical observations in recent ligament ruptures. *Acta Chir Scandi.* 1996;132(6):560-569.
17. Gould N, Seligson D, Gassman J. Early and late repair of lateral ligament of the ankle. *Foot Ankle.* 1980;1(2):84-89.
18. Rosenbaum D, Becker H, Sterk J, Gerngross H, Claes L. Functional evaluation of the 10-year outcome after modified Evans repair for chronic ankle instability. *Foot Ankle Int.* 1997;18(12):765-771.
19. Taranow WS, Conti SF. Surgical treatment of lateral ankle instability. *Operative Tech Ortho.* 1995;5(3):284-289.
20. Coughlin MJ, Schenck RC Jr. Lateral ankle reconstruction. *Foot Ankle Int.* 2001;22(3):256-258.

5

Peroneal Tendon Pathology

James Meeker, MD; Joshua N. Tennant, MD, MPH; and Selene G. Parekh, MD, MBA

Introduction

Peroneal tendon disorders are a significant but often under-diagnosed source of lateral ankle pain. The history of ankle sprain, from which up to 40% of individuals can experience chronic ankle pain, should prompt consideration of peroneal tendon injury and examination of the peroneal anatomy. The 3 primary types of peroneal tendon lesions include tendinitis and tenosynovitis, tendon subluxation and dislocation, and tendon tears and ruptures. The disorder is more common than realized, often overlooked, and can be difficult to differentiate from lateral ankle ligament pathology. In a study by Dombek

Hurwitz SR, Parekh SG. *Musculoskeletal Examination of the Foot and Ankle: Making the Complex Simple* (pp. 78-106).

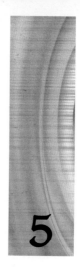

et al,[1] only 60% (24 of 40) of peroneal tendon lesions were correctly diagnosed at the first clinical evaluation.

Typically, peroneal conditions respond to nonoperative treatment such as physical therapy, use of nonsteroidal anti-inflammatory drugs, and immobilization. The literature for operative treatment of peroneal lesions consists largely of case reports and expert opinion. In cases of untreated or under-treated peroneal tendon injuries, persistent lateral ankle pain and substantial functional problems can result.

HISTORY

Peroneal tendinitis or tenosynovitis typically presents following a history of prolonged or repetitive activity, especially after deconditioning from a period of inactivity. Runners, ballet dancers, and individuals with chronic lateral ankle instability are commonly affected, with other causes including severe ankle sprains, fractures of the ankle or calcaneus, and peroneal tubercle hypertrophy or osseous calcaneal tunnel.[2,3] In patients with chronic lateral ankle instability, up to 77% of patients (47 of 61) have been found to have tendinitis or tenosynovitis.[4] Pain, swelling, and point tenderness over the peroneal tendons at the posterolateral aspect of the ankle can be included in the symptoms described by affected patients. *Painful os peroneum syndrome* (POPS) is a term first used by Sobel et al[5] to denote a category of post-traumatic peroneal tendon disorders. The syndrome includes one of the following: 1) an acute fracture of the os peroneum (OP) or diastasis of a multipartite OP, 2) a chronic fracture of the OP associated with stenosing tenosynovitis of the peroneus longus (PL), 3) partial or complete rupture of the PL tendon near the OP, or 4) entrapment of the PL tendon and the OP by a hypertrophied peroneal tubercle.

Peroneal tendon subluxation and dislocation, first described in a ballet dancer in 1803,[6] occur with the displacement of one or both tendons from the retromalleolar groove during tendon loading (Figure 5-1). These can be differentiated as acute or chronic injuries. Tear or attenuation of the superior peroneal retinaculum (SPR) is often associated with the injury. Sudden, reflexive contraction of the peroneal muscles either during

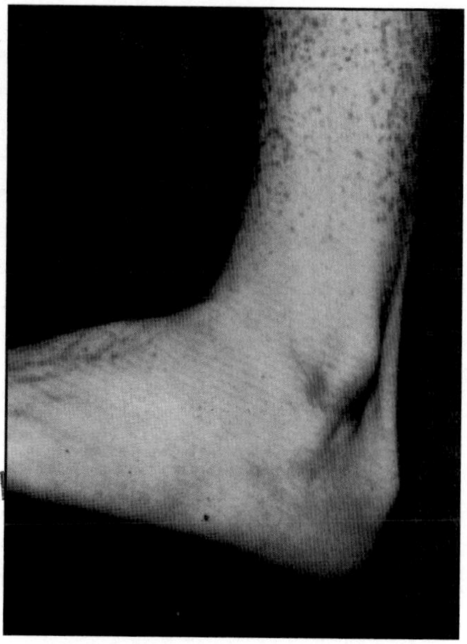

Figure 5-1. Peroneal tendon subluxation. Subluxation of peroneal tendons is visible through the skin. (Martens MA, Noyez JF, Mulier JC. *Am J Sports Med.* 14(2), pp. 148-150, copyright © 1986 by SAGE Publications. Reprinted by Permission of SAGE Publications.)

an acute inversion injury to the dorsiflexed ankle or during forced dorsiflexion of the everted foot[2] are the most common mechanisms, such as the cutting maneuvers that occur during sports like football, soccer, and skiing.[7,8] Injured patients who often report a previous ankle injury may also describe a snapping, popping, or giving way in the ankle.

Peroneal tendon tears are most often associated with acute ankle inversion injuries. A detailed history should include the presence of associated conditions. History usually reveals either an acute traumatic event or a slow, progressive, insidious course of symptoms. Rheumatoid arthritis, psoriasis, hyperparathyroidism, diabetic neuropathy, calcaneal fracture, tophaceous gout, fluoroquinolone use, and local steroid injections have all been reported to increase the prevalence of peroneal tendon tear or dysfunction.[9-15] Isolated peroneal tendon tears and ruptures are rare, and most result from ankle inversion injuries.[16-18] It is also possible that attritional peroneal tendon tears can occur with chronic conditions such as lateral ankle instability, peroneal tendon subluxation, cavovarus foot position, and anatomic variations that lead to stenosis within the retromalleolar groove.[8,19-22] Patients with a peroneus brevis (PB) tear may give a history of a specific traumatic event, repeated ankle sprains, failure to improve after treatment for tenosynovitis, and chronic lateral ankle pain and swelling. Tears of the PL are uncommon. Ankle instability, hindfoot varus, and a hypertrophied peroneal tubercle may also cause PL tears, although they are most commonly related to direct trauma or sports injury.

The diagnosis and treatment of concomitant tears of both peroneal tendons is a relatively new topic, with relatively little having been written about these injuries in the current literature. Steroid injection, diabetes mellitus, rheumatoid arthritis, and injuries associated with peroneal tendon subluxation, dislocation, and instability can all lead to the injury. Tears of both peroneal tendons have been reported in up to 38% (28 of 73) of patients treated operatively for peroneal tendon tears.[23] A retrospective study found a PB tear in 88% and a PL tear in 13% of patients treated operatively for a peroneal tendon tear(s).[1]

Examination

A complete, well-organized history and physical examination of the affected foot and ankle, as well as of the contralateral foot and ankle, are essential for identifying peroneal tendon pathology. Patients with peroneal tendinitis have pain posterior or distal to the lateral malleolus along the course of the peroneal tendons, which is exacerbated by passive hindfoot inversion and ankle plantar flexion or by active-resisted hindfoot eversion and ankle dorsiflexion. When the examiner palpates the course of the peroneal tendons posterior and distal to the distal fibula, tenderness and possible thickening of the tendon is encountered. Acute peroneal tendinitis also has associated swelling and warmth along the tendon sheath. Examination of hindfoot and forefoot alignment should be included because peroneal tendon disorders are more frequently associated with a cavovarus foot. Specific attention should be given to the hindfoot in both static and dynamic positioning, including the Coleman block test if indicated for determining the source of a cavovarus foot deformity (Figure 5-2).[24]

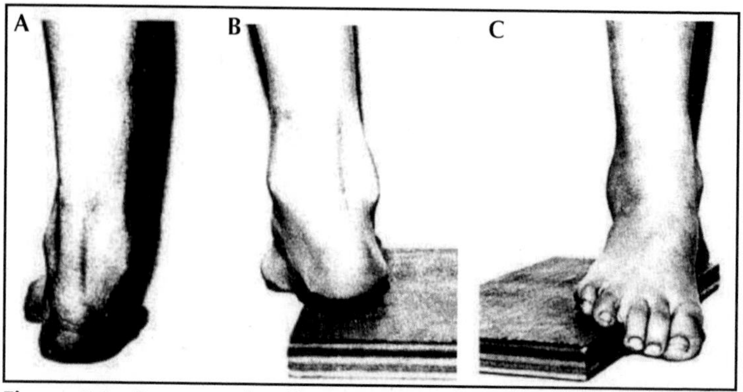

Figure 5-2. Cavovarus hindfoot. The images demonstrate from left to right: (A) varus hindfoot, (B) correction of varus on the block, and (C) plantar flexion of the first ray. (Reprinted with permission of Coleman SS, Chesnut WJ. A simple test for hindfoot flexibility in the cavovarus foot. *Clin Orthop Relat Res.* 1977;(123):60-62.)

A portion of the physical examination can be performed with the patient prone and the knees flexed 90 degrees. Active dorsiflexion and eversion of the ankle or circumduction of the foot generally elicits painful dynamic tendon instability.[2] Palpable snapping or crepitus of the tendons may be evident during these maneuvers. Substantial swelling, tenderness, and ecchymosis are often present posterior to the lateral malleolus in patients with acute peroneal tendon subluxation. Peroneal muscle strength is usually normal when subluxating tendons that are not torn. Concomitant lateral ankle instability is indicated by a positive anterior drawer or talar tilt test.

Peroneal tendon tears are typically accompanied by severe posterolateral ankle pain and swelling along the peroneal tendon sheath.[22,25] Pain may also be present in the cuboid groove or on the plantar aspect of the foot with PL tears. On examination, tenderness and swelling over the tendon sheath are consistent findings, and peroneal muscle strength is often decreased. Loss or limitation of eversion may indicate a peroneus tear. PB tears can be evaluated with the peroneal tunnel compression test.[22] This maneuver involves applying manual pressure along the peroneal tendon sheath in the retromalleolar groove with the knee flexed 90 degrees and the foot plantarflexed. A bulbous pseudotumor in the area of the PB may

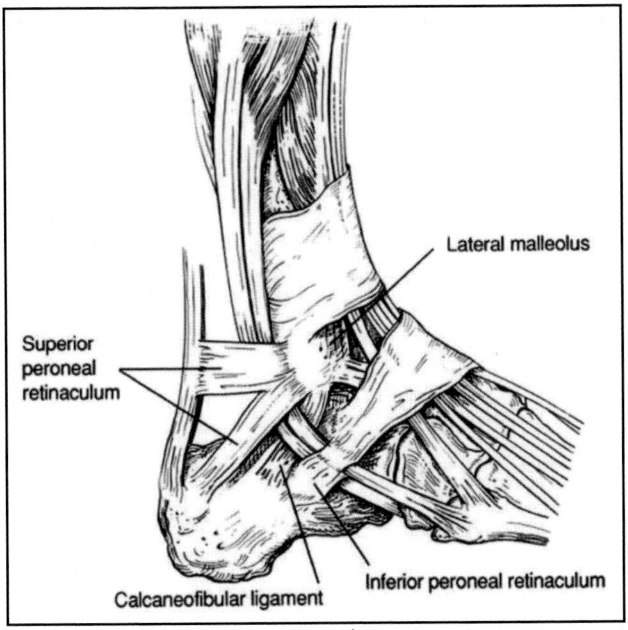

Figure 5-3. Artistic rendering of peroneal tendons. (Reprinted with permission of Shawen S. Indirect groove deepening in the management of chronic peroneal tendon dislocation. *Techniques in Foot and Ankle Surgery.* 2004;3(2):118-125.)

aid in diagnosis,[26] as well as a diagnostic bupivacaine injection into the sheath.[27]

PATHOANATOMY

The PL and PB muscles are located in the lateral compartment of the leg and are innervated by the superficial peroneal nerve, a branch of the common peroneal nerve. The PL originates from the lateral condyle of the tibia and the head of the fibula, coursing down the spiral twist of the fibula, becoming lateral at midtibia. The PB originates from the middle third of the fibula and the intermuscular septum. The PL tendon lies posterolateral to the PB tendon at the level of the lateral malleolus (Figure 5-3).[28] Together, the peroneal tendons provide supplemental lateral ankle stability, especially during the midstance and heel-raise portions of gait. The PB abducts and everts the foot and plantarflexes the ankle, antagonizing the posterior tibialis. The PL everts the foot, plantarflexes the first ray, functions as a secondary plantar flexor of the ankle, and stabilizes the medial column of the foot during stance, antagonizing the flexor hallucis longus, flexor digitorum longus (FDL), and anterior tibialis muscles. Together, the peroneal muscles provide 63% of the total hindfoot eversion strength, with 35% from the PL and 28% from the PB. They are only secondary plantar flexors, making up 4% of the total plantar flexion strength compared with 87% yielded by the gastrocnemius and soleus.[29]

Both peroneal tendons enter a common synovial sheath approximately 4 cm proximal to the tip of the lateral malleolus, running posterior to the lateral malleolus through the retromalleolar groove. This fibro-osseous tunnel, which varies in depth and shape, is formed by the SPR posterolaterally, the fibula anteriorly, and the posterior talofibular, calcaneofibular, and posterior-inferior tibiofibular ligaments medially.[28] The SPR is a fibrous band of tissue 1 to 2 cm wide that serves as the primary restraint to peroneal tendon subluxation at the ankle. Five variations of insertion of the SPR have been described, with the most common type (47% [14 of 30] of cadaver specimens) being a superior band that inserts on the anterior aspect of the Achilles tendon sheath and an inferior band that inserts on the lateral aspect of the calcaneus at the peroneal tubercle.[30] The retromalleolar sulcus is the normal site of PB tears, suggesting mechanical trauma from the contact stresses between tendon and groove. As this typically concave sulcus courses down the posterior aspect of the distal fibula, it measures on average a width of 5 to 10 mm and a depth up to 3 mm.[31] But a lack of concavity along its course, as seen in a cadaveric study, may diminish the stability normally conferred by the groove and predispose the tendons to dislocation, including an 11% absence and a 7% convexity of the fibular groove among 178 specimens.[32] Additional stability to the tendons beyond the fibular groove is provided by a fibrocartilaginous rim, which deepens the groove by 2 to 4 mm.[33]

Distal to the ankle and along the lateral aspect of the calcaneus, the tendon sheath bifurcates around the peroneal tubercle. Both tendons pass through the inferior peroneal

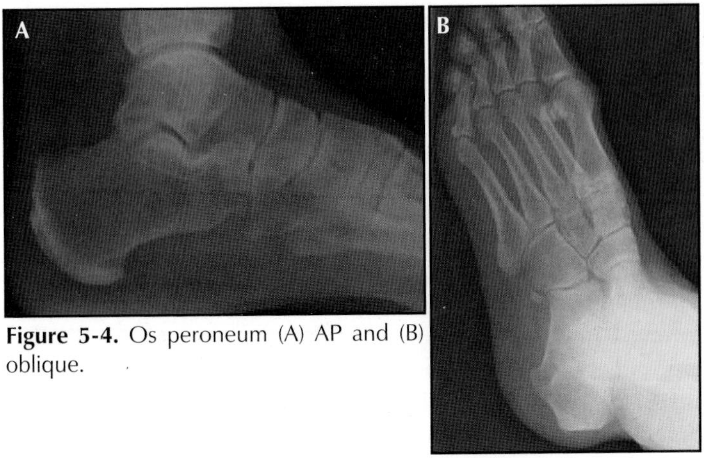

Figure 5-4. Os peroneum (A) AP and (B) oblique.

retinaculum 2 to 3 cm distal to the tip of the fibula. As the PL turns medially, the PB tendon inserts directly onto the fifth metatarsal base tuberosity. In less than 1% of the population, the os vesalianum pedis, an ossicle that can be confused with an acute fracture of the fifth metatarsal base, is found here. The PL tendon courses medially between the cuboid groove and the long plantar ligament toward its insertion onto the plantar surface of the base of the first metatarsal and the lateral aspect of the medial cuneiform.[31] At the level of the calcaneocuboid joint, the OP may be found within the substance of the PL tendon, with prevalence as high as 20% in the general population (Figure 5-4).[34] PL tears usually occur where high shear stresses exist, including the cuboid tunnel, at the OP, at the peroneal tubercle, or at the tip of the lateral malleolus.[35]

The blood supply of the peroneal tendons arises through vincula from the posterior peroneal artery and the medial tarsal artery.[36] Distinct avascular zones have been identified that may contribute to tendinopathy.[8] Petersen et al[37] described 3 distinct avascular zones: 1) in the PB tendon at the turn around the lateral malleolus, 2) in the PL extending from the turn around the lateral malleolus, and 3) another in the PL where the tendon curves around the cuboid. The most common locations of peroneal tendinopathy occur at these watershed avascular zones. However, the presence of peroneal tendon avascular zones have been refuted by other authors,[36] causing the topic to remain controversial.

Several anatomic variations are thought to predispose to peroneal tendon disorders. As noted above, a shallow or narrow retromalleolar groove may affect the stability of the peroneal tendons as they pass posterior to the fibula. By increasing stenosis in the retrofibular groove, either a low-lying PB muscle belly[3] or an accessory peroneus quartus muscle[38] can increase the risk of peroneal tendon injury. The prevalence of the peroneus quartus muscle is between 10% and 22%, and it most often originates from the PB muscle belly and inserts onto the peroneal tubercle of the calcaneus.[39,40] Peroneal tubercle hypertrophy increases friction on the peroneal tendons, potentially leading to tendon injury and restriction of smooth gliding within its sheath.[35] Lastly, a cavovarus hindfoot increases mechanical stress and therefore risk of injury for the peroneal tendons at the lateral malleolus, peroneal tubercle, and cuboid notch.[29]

Imaging

A thorough evaluation of lateral ankle pain requires weight-bearing radiographs of the ankle and foot. Radiographs can detect acute osseous injuries, such as calcaneal fractures, lateral malleolar injury, and the presence of an OP. A Harris heel series may also reveal osseous impingement, hypertrophy of the peroneal tubercle (peroneal process), and spurring of the retromalleolar groove.

Ultrasonography has gained popularity in the evaluation of peroneal tendon disorders. It is relatively inexpensive and noninvasive and does not expose patients to ionizing radiation. Ultrasound is particularly useful in detecting tendon pathology, including peritendinous fluid, tears, ruptures, and thickening. Limitations of ultrasonography include technician proficiency and a significant learning curve.

Three-dimensional imaging helps define the anatomy. Computed tomography (CT) shows osseous architecture and can demonstrate mechanical impingement of the peroneal tendons. Magnetic resonance imaging (MRI) sheds light on the soft tissues and is useful especially in instances of trauma,

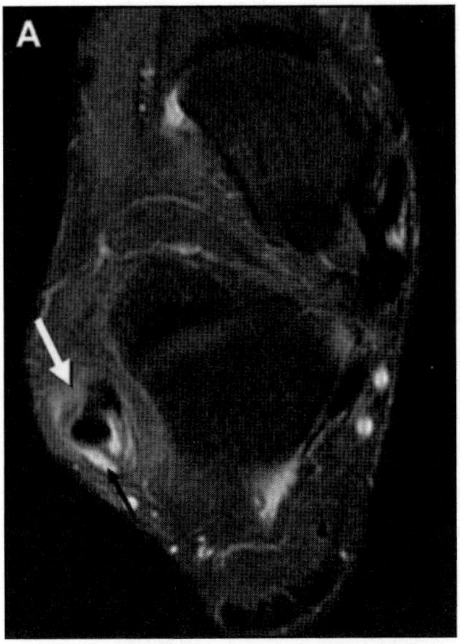

Figure 5-5. Fluid in peroneal tendon sheath demonstrated by MRI. Axial sagittal fat-saturated, intermediate-weighted, fast spin-echo image. The white arrow demonstrates a split tear of the PB tendon. The black arrow shows the surrounding peroneal tenosynovitis caused by peroneal tendon injury. (Reprinted from *Magn Reson Imaging Clin N Am.* 16(1). Collins MS. Imaging evaluation of chronic ankle and hindfoot pain in athletes. 39-58, v-vi. Copyright [2008], with permission from Elsevier.)

masses, arthritis inflammation, and infection. Tendons appear dark on both T1- and T2-weighted images; tendinopathy generally manifests as an altered signal within the body of the tendon.

Tendinitis

Cases of isolated peroneal tendinitis may have causative factors visible on plain film and CT, including osseous impingement. The surest imaging study to confirm tendinitis is MRI. This will show altered signal within the body of the tendon and is often accompanied by fluid-weighted signal within the tenosynovium (Figure 5-5).

Lateral Impingement

Lateral impingement may arise from multiple causes including calcaneal fracture[14] and a prominent peroneal tubercle; both can lead to tendinopathy.[14,41,42] Heel views can be particularly helpful in establishing causes of bony impingement. CT will show the 3-dimensional representation of involved structures especially in instances of post-traumatic deformity (eg, calcaneal fractures) (Figure 5-6).

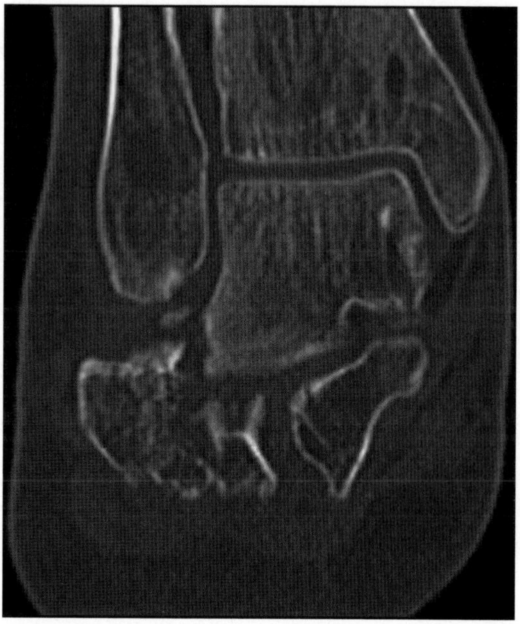

Figure 5-6. CT of lateral impingement. Coronal CT image shows a calcaneal fracture with lateral displacement of fracture fragments into the lateral retromalleolar groove.

Peroneal Tendon Tears

Diagnosing longitudinal tears of peroneal tendons often requires MRI or ultrasonography. When a peroneal tendon tear is suspected, ultrasound can be a powerful tool. A prospective study compared ultrasonography with MRI for the diagnosis of peroneal tendon tears and found that ultrasonography had a sensitivity of 100% and a specificity of 90%; this compared favorably to MRI, which had a sensitivity and specificity of 23% and 100%, respectively.[43] Ultrasonography has an advantage diagnostically and from the standpoint of economic burden to the health care system. However, clinical situations often lead practitioners to order MRI since it offers a superior view of 3-dimensional anatomy.

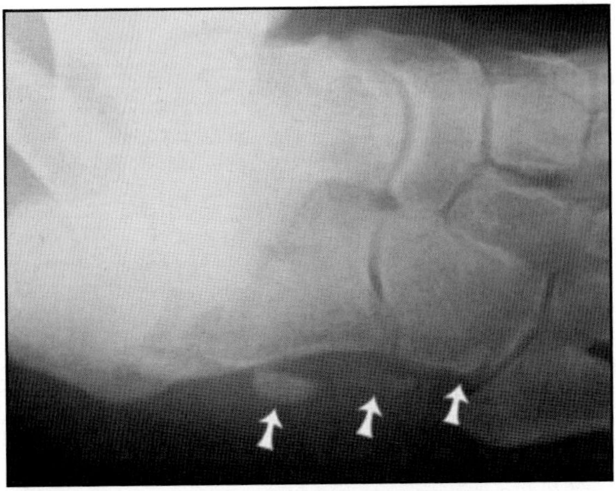

Figure 5-7. OP fracture fragments indicated by arrows. (Reprinted with permission of Brigido MK, Fessell DP, Jacobson JA, et al. Radiography and US of os peroneum fractures and associated peroneal tendon injuries: initial experience. *Radiology*. 2005;237(1):235-41. Radiological Society of North America.)

Acute Ruptures

Acute ruptures of peroneal tendons may occur at osseous interfaces—the OP in the case of the longus and the base of the fifth metatarsal for the brevis. In cases of os fracture, displacement of 1 fragment proximally indicates insufficiency of the PL tendon. Similarly, PL tendon rupture distal to the os results in proximal migration of the entire os (Figure 5-7). Painful degenerative changes of the OP may be detectable on bone scan, but more frequently MRI will be useful to evaluate the condition of the tendon. Careful radiographic examination of the base of the fifth metatarsal can reveal PB insertional pathology. It is important to distinguish between accessory ossicles and avulsion fractures at the base of the fifth metatarsal. An accessory, well-corticated ossicle, termed the *os vesalianum* may reside at the base of the fifth metatarsal.[44]

Peroneal Subluxation

Imaging of peroneal subluxation manifests in a variety of ways. Plain radiographs can be useful in certain situations. The

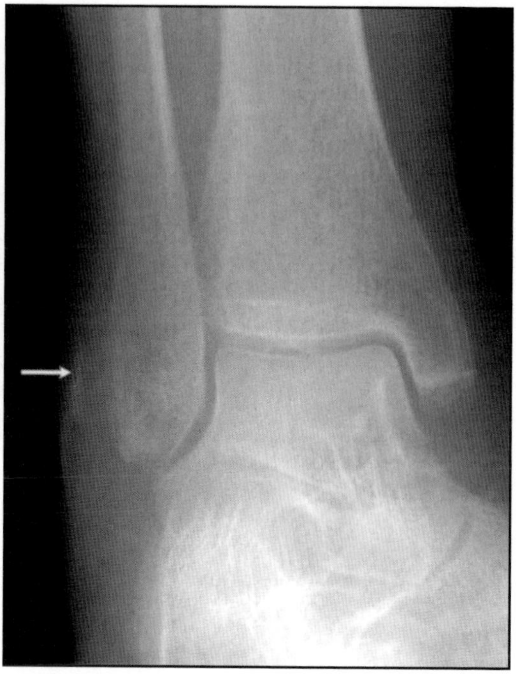

Figure 5-8. Lateral malleolar fleck. The arrow points to avulsed fibular fibro-osseous attachment of the SPR. (Copyright © 2011 by the American Orthopaedic Foot and Ankle Society, Inc., originally published in *Foot & Ankle International*, 2007;28(1):49-54 and reproduced here with permission.)

presence of an osseous fleck above the malleolus often indicates an avulsion injury to the SPR (Figure 5-8).[45] More frequently, peroneal subluxation presents with soft tissue disruption. One study has classified the morphology of the lateral malleolar groove as concave, flat, or convex, but found no correlation between malleolar shape and dislocation.[46] However, it should be noted that a more shallow malleolar groove provides less restraint to subluxation than one that cups the tendons. The role of cross-sectional imaging in cases of peroneal instability is somewhat controversial. The tendons usually lie in a subcutaneous position, and subluxation is visually apparent (see Figure 5-1). However, in cases of acute trauma with swelling or significant obesity, MRI may be required to make a diagnosis (Figure 5-9). Ultrasound offers real-time imaging and can identify episodic peroneal subluxation in cases where there is question. The positive predictive value of this modality is reported to be 100%.[47] Ultrasound is used with increased frequency in the office setting but is limited by the need for operator proficiency (Table 5-1).

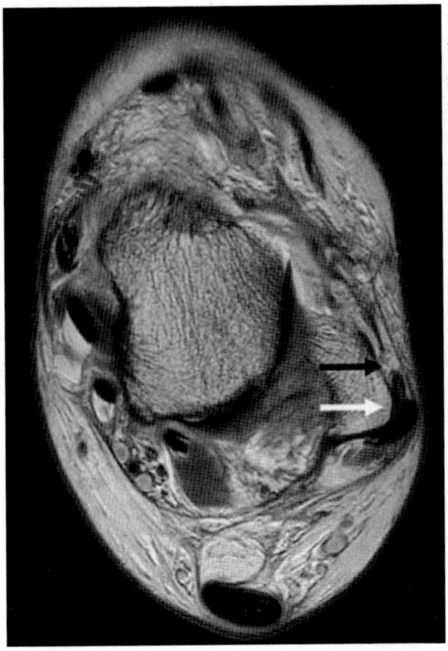

Figure 5-9. MRI of dislocated tendons. Axial proton density image of both peroneal tendons subluxated from the retromalleolar groove (white arrow). The black arrow indicates the avulsed cartilaginous portion of the retromalleolar groove. (Reprinted from *Magn Reson Imaging Clin N Am.* 16(1). Campbell SE, Warner M. MR imaging of ankle inversion injuries. 1-18, v. Copyright [2008] with permission from Elsevier.)

Treatment

Tendinitis

Peroneal tendinitis can present as a primary condition but is often associated with other ankle pathology. Prior to entertaining operative treatment, conservative measures ought to be exhausted. A period of rest, ice, elevation, and activity modification along with therapeutic modalities should be undertaken. A brief period of immobilization may also allow for symptomatic recovery. Systemic and transdermal nonsteroidal anti-inflammatories may ameliorate symptoms. Injections of corticosteroid and other adjunctive agents have yielded mixed results in the setting of tendinopathy, and there is concern that steroid injection may predispose the patient to tendon rupture.[48,49] Platelet-rich plasma has unproven effects but may advance the process of tendon healing. The initial treatment in peroneal tendinitis should consist of conservative measures; when this is unsuccessful, operative treatment is considered.

Table 5-1

Methods for Examining Peroneal Tendon Pathology

	Clinical Presentation	*X-Ray Finding*	*CT Finding*	*MRI Finding*
PB longitudinal tear	Lateral pain	None	None	Signal change within the substance of the tendon
PB rupture	Eversion weakness and pain	None; base of the fifth avulsion	Base of the fifth MT avulsion	Rupture of the PB tendon; injury to the base of the fifth MT
Peroneal tendon subluxation	Lateral pain with eversion	None; osteochondral avulsion from the lateral malleolus (fleck)	None; avulsion (fleck); flattening of peroneal groove	Rupture of SPR; osteochondral avulsion
Peroneal tendonitis	Pain with range of motion	None	None	Signal change within the substance of the tendon; fluid within the tendon sheath

Refractory cases of peroneal tendinitis merit operative consideration. This involves open tendon débridement and tenosynovectomy. A lateral incision begins 1 cm posterior to the tip of the fibula, follows the course of the peroneals, and may be extended to the brevis insertion on the base of the fifth metatarsal. During the approach, use caution to avoid injury to the sural nerve, which courses through the retromalleolar area between the lateral malleolus and the tendo Achilles (Figure 5-10); it then advances distally inferior to, then passing over,

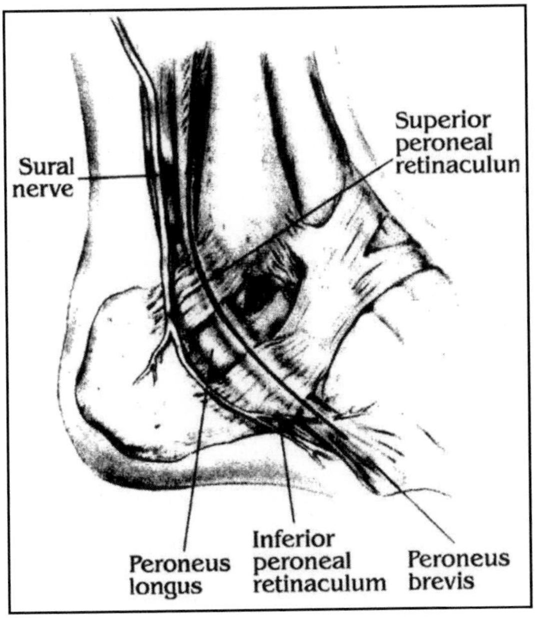

Figure 5-10. Sural nerve. (Copyright © 2011 by the American Orthopaedic Foot and Ankle Society, Inc., originally published in *Foot & Ankle International*, 2000;21(10):809-815 and reproduced here with permission.)

the peroneal tendon sheaths. The peroneal tendon sheath is then opened longitudinally to inspect each tendon; débride any areas of inflammatory tissue; excise the peroneus quartus (or low lying brevis) muscle if it is present. Exploration of the PL tendon should include its passage at the cuboid. If a prominent peroneal tubercle prevents smooth excursion of the tendons (Figure 5-11), consider excision. Look for associated longitudinal tears in both tendons, and repair them using a tubularization technique. Be sure to consider and address any anatomic factors that might contribute to peroneal tendinopathy (ie, cavovarus hindfoot, painful os, and lateral instability).

Longitudinal Tears of the Peroneus Brevis

Longitudinal tears arise most commonly in the PB tendon at the level of the retromalleolar groove (Figure 5-12). After the correct diagnosis is made and conservative measures are exhausted, operative consideration is warranted. Before surgery, be certain to identify any lateral instability, hindfoot malalignment, a prominent peroneal tubercle, and peroneal subluxation; the presence of such factors will

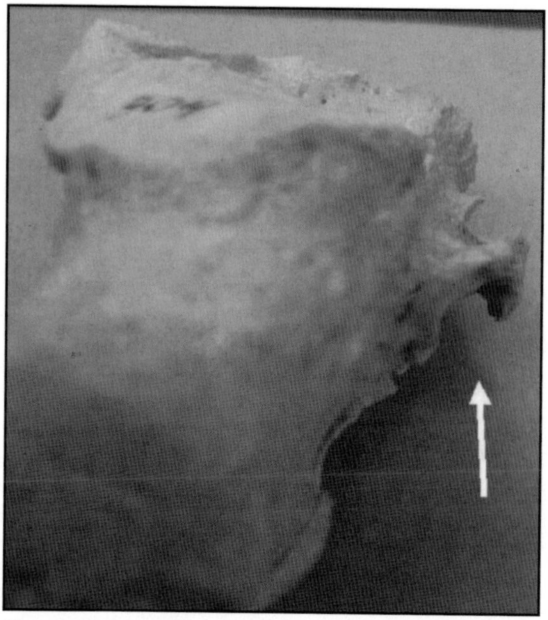

Figure 5-11. Prominent peroneal tubercle. The peroneal tubercle is hypertrophied. The PB passes superiorly, while the longus passes below. (Copyright © 2011 by the American Orthopaedic Foot and Ankle Society, Inc., originally published in *Foot & Ankle International*, 2005;26(11):947-950 and reproduced here with permission.)

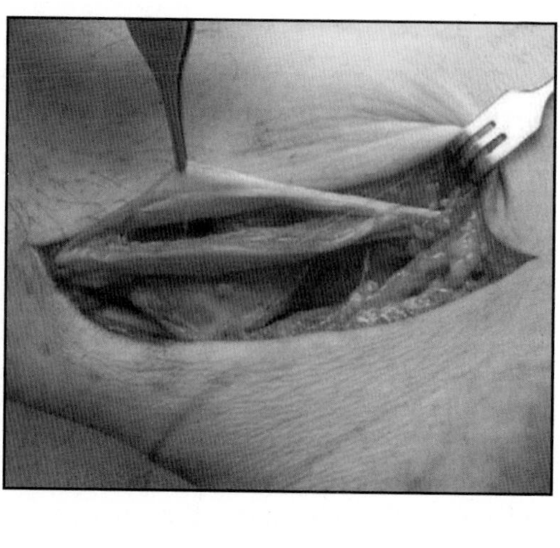

Figure 5-12. PB tear. (Reprinted from *Foot Ankle Clin.* Squires. 12(4). N, Myerson MS, Gamba C. Surgical treatment of peroneal tendon tears. 675-95, vii. Copyright [2007] with permission from Elsevier.)

Table 5-2

TECHNICAL TRICKS IN WORKING WITH THE PERONEAL TENDONS

- Protect subcutaneous nerves (superficial peroneal and sural).
- When opening the peroneal tendon sheaths, leave a 3- to 5-mm cuff of superficial peroneal retinacular tissue for later repair.
- Examine both tendons for injuries. Assess whether or not repair is appropriate.
- Consider other factors that may contribute to peroneal dysfunction such as hindfoot alignment and ankle instability. Address these factors at the time of surgery.
- Avoid overstuffing the retromalleolar groove. Avoid tenodesis within 3 to 5 cm of the retromalleolar groove. Excise low-lying and accessory muscles.
- During closure of the SPR, reef any redundant tissue using pants over vest technique, but avoid creating a point of stenosis.

alter surgical management. The most common cause of poor outcome in peroneal tendon surgery is failure to correctly identify causative pathology (Table 5-2).[28]

Simple longitudinal tears may be treated with tubularization (Figure 5-13) to permit more smooth tendon excursion. Approach the peroneal tendons with a lateral extensile incision, curving posterior and distal to the lateral malleolus. The superficial peroneal nerve is at risk above the malleolus and the sural nerve may be injured below. Identify and incise the SPR. Preserve a 3- to 5-mm cuff of this tissue for later repair. Examine each tendon for tears, degenerative changes, and inflammation; perform débridement as appropriate. If 50% of healthy tendon cross-sectional area remains, proceed with tubularization.[25] Tubularization consists of using 3-0 or 4-0 suture on both the deep and superficial sides of the tear (Figure 5-13). If a peroneus quartus or low-lying brevis muscle is present, excise them to prevent overstuffing of the retromalleolar groove.[50] In cases where more than half of the tendon's cross-sectional area is débrided, the tendon's strength is

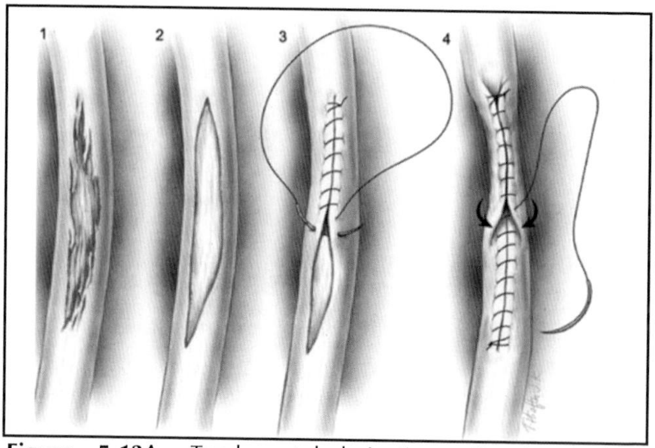

Figure 5-13A. Tendon tubularization. (Reprinted from *Arthroscopy,* 25(11), Bare A, Ferkel RD, Peroneal tendon tears: associated arthroscopic findings and results after repair. 1288-1297, 2009 with permission from Elsevier.)

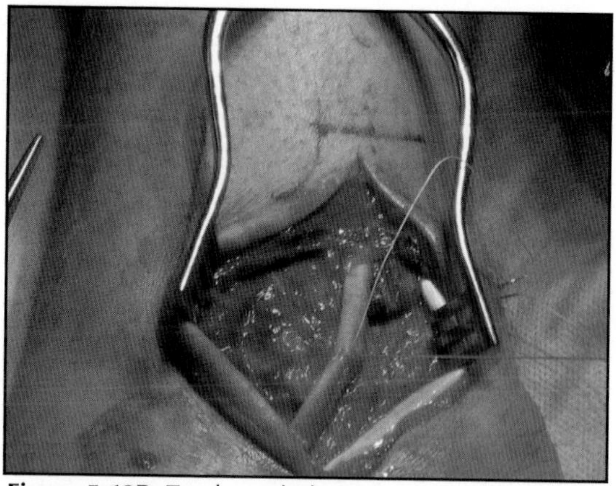

Figure 5-13B. Tendon tubularization. (Reprinted with permission of Selene G. Parekh.)

sufficiently weakened to require a different procedure. Depending on the situation, consider tenodesis, autograft augmentation, tendon transfer, or allograft reconstruction.[15]

Peroneus Longus Tendinopathy

The PL tendon is subject to different pathology from the PB. While the longus can be subject to longitudinal tears, it is more likely to suffer from attritional tears at the level of the peroneal tubercle and cuboid groove. PL tendinopathy has a strong association with cavovarus foot deformity.[20] Acute PL tenosynovitis in athletes is often successfully treated with a period of rest, conservative measures, and modified training habits.[51] However, when the PL sustains chronic irritation and injury, then operative intervention may be warranted. Important presurgical planning involves assessment of hindfoot alignment, ankle stability, evidence of peroneal tubercle hypertrophy, presence of an OP, retinacular insufficiency, and injury to the PB tendon.

Cases of PL tendon longitudinal tears may be treated with débridement and tubularization provided that adequate healthy tendon remains. This is performed in a similar manner to the repair of PB tendons. The causative factors in the tendon tear ought to be addressed at the time of surgery. Hindfoot malalignment, ankle instability, and tendon instability should be corrected. Also, an enlarged, degenerative peroneal tubercle ought to be removed to improve tendon excursion.[52,53]

Peroneal Instability

Peroneal instability may arise from a variety of causes, including trauma, hindfoot alignment, and anatomic factors. The instability may even be subtle, presenting merely as pain and mechanical symptoms.[54,55] Once instability is diagnosed, it is important to address any underlying causative factors when planning treatment. Acute injuries have been treated with initial conservative measures, including heel lifts, taping, orthotics, and often cast immobilization.[56-58] Results of this treatment are inconsistent, and as many as 75% of patients experience limited improvement.[7] Recurrent episodes of subluxation or redislocation can lead to tearing of the PB tendon. Therefore, one ought to strongly consider acute surgical repair. The variants of injury to the superior retinacular ligament have been described by Eckert and Davis.[59] Numerous surgical procedures have been described to stabilize the tendons in the lateral malleolar groove.[59,60-62] Anatomic factors that

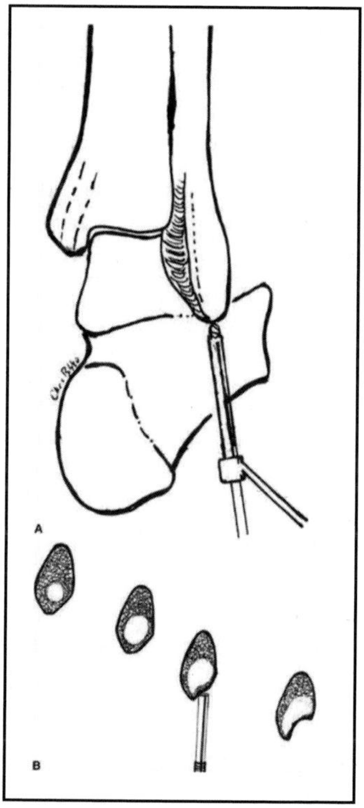

Figure 5-14. (A, B) Groove deepening. (Reprinted with permission of Shawen S, Anderson R. Indirect groove deepening in the management of chronic peroneal tendon dislocation. *Techniques in Foot and Ankle Surgery*. 2004;3(2):118-125.)

predispose dislocation such as a shallow retromalleolar groove should be addressed at the time of surgery.[63] Peroneal tendon subluxation may arise in conjunction with other predisposing factors such as lateral ankle instability.[7] In instances of peroneal tendon dislocation associated with fracture in the hindfoot or ankle, percutaneous stabilization of the tendons has been described.[64]

There are numerous methods of stabilizing the peroneal tendons. The general goal in addressing peroneal instability involves providing a smooth gliding track for tendon excursion and preventing tendon subluxation. Key features of surgical management should include careful examination of the tendons and treatment of any injury when present. To achieve stability, the most common current practices involve deepening the retromalleolar groove through one of several techniques (Figure 5-14).[65-67] Since it is also common to see

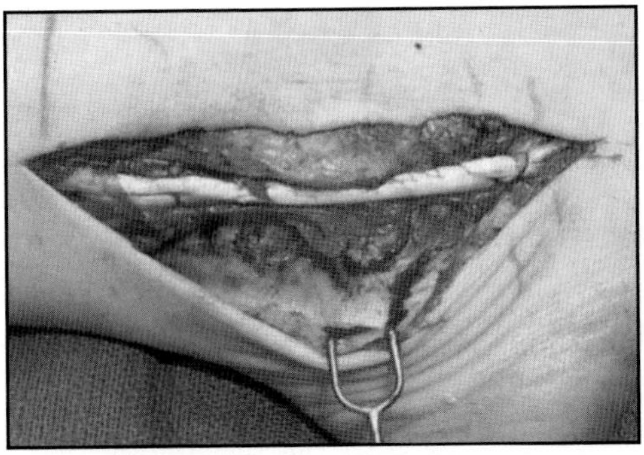

Figure 5-15. Tenodesis of brevis to longus. (Copyright © 2011 by the American Orthopaedic Foot and Ankle Society, Inc., originally published in *Foot & Ankle International*, 2004;25(10):695-707 and reproduced here with permission.)

insufficiency of the superior retinacular ligament, a reefing procedure ought to be performed to hold the tendons in the groove without creating a stenotic passage.

Irreparable Peroneal Tendon Injuries

Chronic irreparable injury to one or both peroneal tendons may necessitate tenodesis or reconstruction. Redfern and Myerson developed an algorithm with treatment recommendations depending on the degree of tendon pathology.[23] For example, when the PL tendon is deemed unsuitable for repair, but the PB is viable, tenodesis may be performed after excising the diseased portion of the tendon. In the converse, when the PB is irreparably damaged (>50% loss of cross-sectional area) then tenodesis to the longus may be performed (Figure 5-15). In this case, it is advisable also to section the longus at the cuboid tunnel and perform anastomosis to the distal brevis stump; this reduces the plantar flexion imbalance.[68] When performing tenodesis, use 2-0 nonabsorbable suture over at least 2 cm of tendon length.[69] Avoid anastomoses in proximity to the retromalleolar groove; stay 3 cm above and 5 cm below the groove to allow for adequate excursion.[25]

When neither tendon is viable for tenodesis, tendon transfer and reconstruction may be considered. Redfern and Myerson identified 2 intraoperative factors that are critical for decision making: musculotendinous excursion and viability of the tendon sheath. The tendon sheath must be sufficiently free of scar tissue to permit smooth passage of tendon. In absence of this, staged procedures can be performed using Hunter rods

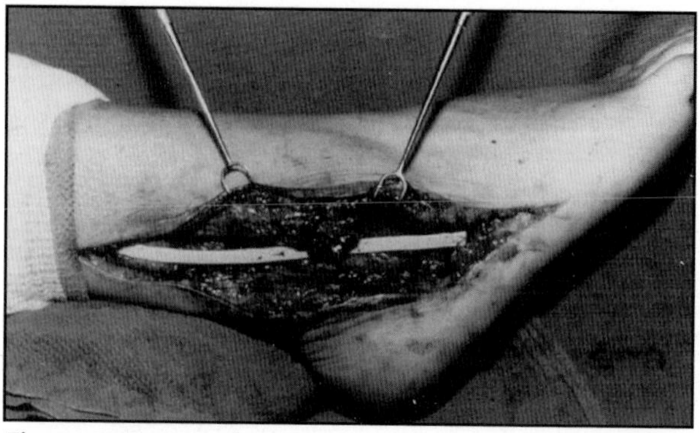

Figure 5-16. Staged peroneal reconstruction using Hunter rods. (Copyright © 2011 by the American Orthopaedic Foot and Ankle Society, Inc., originally published in *Foot & Ankle International*, 2006;27(8):591-597 and reproduced here with permission.)

(Figure 5-16).[70,71] The decision from this point hinges upon the adequacy of proximal musculotendinous excursion. When the musculotendinous unit is free of scarring and remains functional, it is amenable to reconstruction with allograft tendon.[23] However, when the native peroneal musculature is no longer functional, consider FDL transfer to the distal stump of the brevis.[72] It is noteworthy that authors have advocated the use of platelet-rich plasma in the setting of tendon healing.[73,74] Others have reported successful treatment of irreparable injuries to the peroneal tendons with acellular dermal matrix used to augment repair.[75] It remains to be seen what role these adjuncts will have in tendon repair and reconstruction.

OP disorders fall into a spectrum where treatment depends on pathology. Acute rupture of the PL tendon through a fractured or bipartite OP is rare (Figure 5-17)[76]; successful treatment has been accomplished by excising all or part of the remnant os, and performing end-to-end repair.[5,75] In a different variant, the intact os can become inflamed acutely in the cuboid groove, resulting in pain. In such cases, conservative treatment should include immobilization, orthoses, anti-inflammatories, and consideration of a judiciously placed injection. Cases of chronically painful OP may be better suited to surgical treatment with resection of the sesamoid.

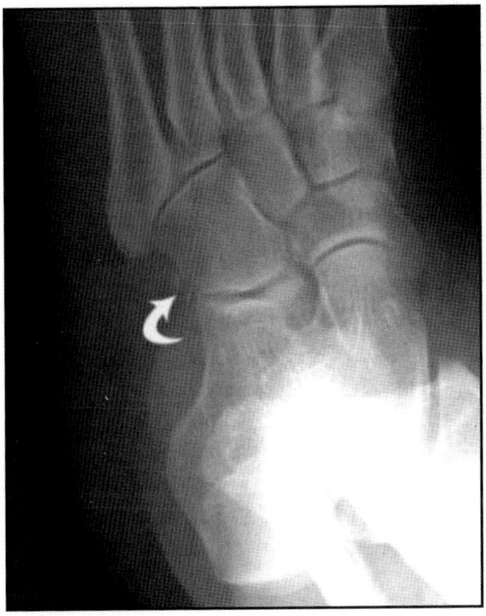

Figure 5-17. Bipartite os. (Reprinted with permission of Brigido MK, Fessell DP, Jacobson JA, et al. Radiography and US of os peroneum fractures and associated peroneal tendon injuries: initial experience. *Radiology.* 2005;237(1):235-241.)

End-to-end tendon repair versus tenodesis should be based on the condition of the host tendon and amount of excursion present.[23] Concomitant factors such as hindfoot varus should be addressed at the time of surgery.

Postoperative protocols involving peroneal tendons will vary somewhat according to the procedure. The goal of most peroneal tendon surgery is to provide a stable, painless, plantigrade foot. The initial 2 weeks after surgery ought to involve immobilization in a short leg splint. This should prevent foot plantar flexion and dorsiflexion to allow for the soft tissues to heal adequately. To relieve stresses placed upon the peroneal tendons, slight immobilization in slight plantar flexion and eversion is encouraged. Protected weight bearing may be permitted during this time if there is no fracture work or concern about complex tendon reconstruction. Early, gentle range of motion is generally encouraged early to prevent tendon sheath fibrosis. Immobilization is usually continued for 6 to 8 weeks, but some form of support may be needed for 3 to 6 months.

Conclusion

Peroneal tendon pathology can manifest itself in a variety of forms. Depending on the type of problem, the symptoms can range from mild to severe. A combination of history, physical examination, and often imaging will lead to a diagnosis. It is particularly important to consider the possibility of concomitant ankle instability when assessing peroneal tendon disorders. If present, instability needs to be addressed to avoid recurrent peroneal tendon problems.

References

1. Dombek MF, Lamm BM, Saltrick K, Mendicino RW, Catanzariti AR. Peroneal tendon tears: a retrospective review. *J Foot Ankle Surg.* 2003 42(5):250-258.
2. Safran MR, O'Malley D,Jr, Fu FH. Peroneal tendon subluxation in athletes: New exam technique, case reports, and review. *Med Sci Sports Exerc.* 1999;31(7)(suppl):S487-492.
3. Geller J, Lin S, Cordas D, Vieira P. Relationship of a low-lying muscle belly to tears of the peroneus brevis tendon. *Am J Orthop.* 2003;32(11):541-544.
4. DiGiovanni BF, Fraga CJ, Cohen BE, Shereff MJ. Associated injuries found in chronic lateral ankle instability. *Foot Ankle Int.* 2000;21(10):809-815.
5. Sobel M, Pavlov H, Geppert MJ, Thompson FM, DiCarlo EF, Davis WH. Painful os peroneum syndrome: A spectrum of conditions responsible for plantar lateral foot pain. *Foot Ankle Int.* 1994;15(3):112-124.
6. Monteggia G. *Instituzioni chirurgiche,* 2nd ed. Milan, Italy: G. Maspero; 1813-1815.
7. Escalas F, Figueras JM, Merino JA. Dislocation of the peroneal tendons. Long-term results of surgical treatment. *J Bone Joint Surg Am.* 1980;62(3):451-453.
8. Sammarco GJ. Peroneus longus tendon tears: acute and chronic. *Foot Ankle Int.* 1995;16(5):245-253.
9. Lagoutaris ED, Adams HB, DiDomenico LA, Rothenberg RJ. Longitudinal tears of both peroneal tendons associated with tophaceous gouty infiltration. A case report. *J Foot Ankle Surg.* 2005;44(3):222-224.
10. Sharma P, Maffulli N. Tendon injury and tendinopathy: healing and repair. *J Bone Joint Surg Am.* 2005;87(1):187-202.
11. Wright DG, Sangeorzan BJ. Calcaneal fracture with peroneal impingement and tendon dysfunction. *Foot Ankle Int.* 1996;17(10):650.
12. Vainio K. The rheumatoid foot. A clinical study with pathological and roentgenological comments. 1956. *Clin Orthop Relat Res.* 1991;(265):4-8.

13. Truong DT, Dussault RG, Kaplan PA. Fracture of the os peroneum and rupture of the peroneus longus tendon as a complication of diabetic neuropathy. *Skeletal Radiol.* 1995;24(8):626-628.
14. Rosenberg ZS, Feldman F, Singson RD, Price GJ. Peroneal tendon injury associated with calcaneal fractures: CT findings. *AJR Am J Roentgenol.* 1987;149(1):125-129.
15. Borton DC, Lucas P, Jomha NM, Cross MJ, Slater K. Operative reconstruction after transverse rupture of the tendons of both peroneus longus and brevis. Surgical reconstruction by transfer of the flexor digitorum longus tendon. *J Bone Joint Surg Br.* 1998;80(5):781-784.
16. Evans JD. Subcutaneous rupture of the tendon of peroneus longus. Report of a case. *J Bone Joint Surg Br.* 1966;48(3):507-509.
17. Davies JA. Peroneal compartment syndrome secondary to rupture of the peroneus longus. A case report. *J Bone Joint Surg Am.* 1979;61(5):783-784.
18. Abraham E, Stirnaman JE. Neglected rupture of the peroneal tendons causing recurrent sprains of the ankle. Case report. *J Bone Joint Surg Am.* 1979;61(8):1247-1248.
19. Sobel M, Geppert MJ, Warren RF. Chronic ankle instability as a cause of peroneal tendon injury. *Clin Orthop Relat Res.* 1993;(296):187-191.
20. Brandes CB, Smith RW. Characterization of patients with primary peroneus longus tendinopathy: a review of twenty-two cases. *Foot Ankle Int.* 2000;21(6):462-468.
21. Bonnin M, Tavernier T, Bouysset M. Split lesions of the peroneus brevis tendon in chronic ankle laxity. *Am J Sports Med.* 1997;25(5):699-703.
22. Sobel M, Geppert MJ, Olson EJ, Bohne WH, Arnoczky SP. The dynamics of peroneus brevis tendon splits: a proposed mechanism, technique of diagnosis, and classification of injury. *Foot Ankle.* 1992;13(7):413-422.
23. Redfern D, Myerson M. The management of concomitant tears of the peroneus longus and brevis tendons. *Foot Ankle Int.* 2004;25(10):695-707.
24. Coleman SS, Chesnut WJ. A simple test for hindfoot flexibility in the cavovarus foot. *Clin Orthop Relat Res.* 1977;(123):60-62.
25. Krause JO, Brodsky JW. Peroneus brevis tendon tears: pathophysiology, surgical reconstruction, and clinical results. *Foot Ankle Int.* 1998;19(5):271-279.
26. Webster FS. Peroneal tenosynovitis with pseudotumor. *J Bone Joint Surg Am.* 1968;50:153-157.
27. Mizel MS, Michelson JD, Newberg A. Peroneal tendon bupivacaine injection: utility of concomitant injection of contrast material. *Foot Ankle Int.* 1996;17(9):566-568.
28. Molloy R, Tisdel C. Failed treatment of peroneal tendon injuries. *Foot Ankle Clin.* 2003;8(1):115-29, ix.
29. Manoli A 2nd, Graham B. The subtle cavus foot, "the underpronator". *Foot Ankle Int.* 2005;26(3):256-263.
30. Davis WH, Sobel M, Deland J, Bohne WH, Patel MB. The superior peroneal retinaculum: an anatomic study. *Foot Ankle Int.* 1994;15(5):271-275.
31. Mann RA, Haskell A. Biomechanics of the foot and ankle. In: *Surgery of the Foot and Ankle*, 8th ed. Philadelphia, PA: Mosby Elsevier; 2007. 3-44.
32. Edwards M. The relations of theperoneal tendons to the fibula, calcaneusand cuboideum. *Am J Anat.* 1928;42:213-253.

33. Kumai T, Benjamin M. The histological structure of the malleolar groove of the fibula in man: its direct bearing on the displacement of peroneal tendons and their surgical repair. *J Anat.* 2003;203(2):257-262.
34. Sobel M, DiCarlo EF, Bohne WH, Collins L. Longitudinal splitting of the peroneus brevis tendon: an anatomic and histologic study of cadaveric material. *Foot Ankle.* 1991;12(3):165-170.
35. Hyer CF, Dawson JM, Philbin TM, Berlet GC, Lee TH. The peroneal tubercle: description, classification, and relevance to peroneus longus tendon pathology. *Foot Ankle Int.* 2005;26(11):947-950.
36. Sobel M, Geppert MJ, Hannafin JA, Bohne WH, Arnoczky SP. Microvascular anatomy of the peroneal tendons. *Foot Ankle.* 1992;13(8):469-472.
37. Petersen W, Bobka T, Stein V, Tillmann B. Blood supply of the peroneal tendons: injection and immunohistochemical studies of cadaver tendons. *Acta Orthop Scand.* 2000;71(2):168-174.
38. Zammit J, Singh D. The peroneus quartus muscle. Anatomy and clinical relevance. *J Bone Joint Surg Br.* 2003;85(8):1134-1137.
39. Cheung YY, Rosenberg ZS, Ramsinghani R, Beltran J, Jahss MH. Peroneus quartus muscle: MR imaging features. *Radiology.* 1997;202(3):745-750.
40. Sobel M, Levy ME, Bohne WH. Congenital variations of the peroneus quartus muscle: an anatomic study. *Foot Ankle.* 1990;11(2):81-89.
41. Sugimoto K, Takakura Y, Okahashi K, Tanaka Y, Ohshima M, Kasanami R. Enlarged peroneal tubercle with peroneus longus tenosynovitis. *J Orthop Sci.* 2009;14(3):330-335.
42. Rademaker J, Rosenberg ZS, Delfaut EM, Cheung YY, Schweitzer ME. Tear of the peroneus longus tendon: MR imaging features in nine patients. *Radiology.* 2000;214(3):700-704.
43. Rockett MS, Waitches G, Sudakoff G, Brage M. Use of ultrasonography versus magnetic resonance imaging for tendon abnormalities around the ankle. *Foot Ankle Int.* 1998;19(9):604-612.
44. Inoue T, Yoshimura I, Ogata K, Emoto G. Os vesalianum as a cause of lateral foot pain: a familial case and its treatment. *J Pediatr Orthop B.* 1999;8(1):56-58.
45. Church CC. Radiographic diagnosis of acute peroneal tendon dislocation. *AJR Am J Roentgenol.* 1977;129(6):1065-1068.
46. Adachi N, Fukuhara K, Kobayashi T, Nakasa T, Ochi M. Morphologic variations of the fibular malleolar groove with recurrent dislocation of the peroneal tendons. *Foot Ankle Int.* 2009;30(6):540-544.
47. Neustadter J, Raikin SM, Nazarian LN. Dynamic sonographic evaluation of peroneal tendon subluxation. *AJR Am J Roentgenol.* 2004;183(4):985-988.
48. Mahler F, Fritschy D. Partial and complete ruptures of the Achilles tendon and local corticosteroid injections. *Br J Sports Med.* 1992;26(1):7-14.
49. Madsen BL, Noer HH. Simultaneous rupture of both peroneal tendons after corticosteroid injection: operative treatment. *Injury* .1999;30(4):299-300.
50. Sobel M, Bohne WH, O'Brien SJ. Peroneal tendon subluxation in a case of anomalous peroneus brevis muscle. *Acta Orthop Scand.* 1992;63(6):682-684.

51. Folan JC. Peroneus longus tenosynovitis. *Br J Sports Med.* 1981;15(4):277-279.
52. Chen YJ, Hsu RW, Huang TJ. Hypertrophic peroneal tubercle with stenosing tenosynovitis: the results of surgical treatment. *Changgeng Yi Xue Za Zhi.* 1998;21(4):442-446.
53. Bruce WD, Christofersen MR, Phillips DL. Stenosing tenosynovitis and impingement of the peroneal tendons associated with hypertrophy of the peroneal tubercle. *Foot Ankle Int.* 1999;20(7):464-467.
54. Raikin SM, Elias I, Nazarian LN. Intrasheath subluxation of the peroneal tendons. *J Bone Joint Surg Am.* 2008;90(5):992-999.
55. Raikin SM. Intrasheath subluxation of the peroneal tendons. Surgical technique. *J Bone Joint Surg Am.* 2009; 91(suppl 2 pt 1):146-155.
56. Ogawa BK, Thordarson DB. Current concepts review: peroneal tendon subluxation and dislocation. *Foot Ankle Int.* 2007;28(9):1034-1040.
57. Sarmiento A, Wolf M. Subluxation of peroneal tendons. Case treated by rerouting tendons under calcaneofibular ligament. *J Bone Joint Surg Am.* 1975;57(1):115-116.
58. Oden RR. Tendon injuries about the ankle resulting from skiing. *Clin Orthop Relat Res.* 1987;(216):63-69.
59. Eckert WR, Davis EA Jr. Acute rupture of the peroneal retinaculum. *J Bone Joint Surg Am.* 1976;58(5):670-672.
60. Marti R. Dislocation of the peroneal tendons. *Am J Sports Med.* 1977;5(1):19-22.
61. Arrowsmith SR, Fleming LL, Allman FL. Traumatic dislocations of the peroneal tendons. *Am J Sports Med.* 1983;11(3):142-146.
62. Murr S. Dislocation of the peroneal tendons with marginal fracture of the lateral malleolus. *JBJS(Br).* 1961;43 B(3):563-565.
63. Brage ME, Hansen ST Jr. Traumatic subluxation/dislocation of the peroneal tendons. *Foot Ankle.* 1992;13(7):423-431.
64. Summers H, Kramer PA, Benirschke SK. Percutaneous stabilization of traumatic peroneal tendon dislocation. *Foot Ankle Int.* 2008;29(12):1229-1231.
65. Shawen S. Indirect groove deepening in the management of chronic peroneal tendon dislocation. *Techniques in Foot and Ankle Surgery.* 2004;3(2):118-125.
66. Kollias SL, Ferkel RD. Fibular grooving for recurrent peroneal tendon subluxation. *Am J Sports Med.* 1997;25(3):329-335.
67. Ogawa BK, Thordarson DB, Zalavras C. Peroneal tendon subluxation repair with an indirect fibular groove deepening technique. *Foot Ankle Int.* 2007;28(11):1194-1197.
68. Cerrato RA. Tenodesis and transfer procedures for peroneal tears and tendinosis. *Techniques in Foot & Ankle Surgery.* 2009;8(3):119-125.
69. Ritter C. Acute peroneal tendon tears. *Techniques in Foot & Ankle Surgery.* 2009;8(3):106-111.
70. Wapner KL, Taras JS, Lin SS, Chao W. Staged reconstruction for chronic rupture of both peroneal tendons using Hunter rod and flexor hallucis longus tendon transfer: a long-term followup study. *Foot Ankle Int.* 2006;27(8):591-597.

71. Wapner K. Reconstruction of chronic peroneal ruptures with staged Hunter rods and a flexor hallucis longus transfer. *Techniques in Foot & Ankle Surgery.* 2005;4(3):202-206.
72. Wapner K. Late peroneal reconstructions using FHL as a primary and staged procedure. *Techniques in Foot & Ankle Surgery.* 2009;8(4):190-193.
73. Sanchez M, Anitua E, Azofra J, Andia I, Padilla S, Mujika I. Comparison of surgically repaired Achilles tendon tears using platelet-rich fibrin matrices. *Am J Sports Med.* 2007;35(2):245-251.
74. Lyras DN, Kazakos K, Verettas D, et al. The influence of platelet-rich plasma on angiogenesis during the early phase of tendon healing. *Foot Ankle Int.* 2009;30(11):1101-1106.
75. Rapley JH, Crates J, Barber A. Mid-substance peroneal tendon defects augmented with an acellular dermal matrix allograft. *Foot Ankle Int.* 2010;31(2):136-140.
76. Patterson MJ, Cox WK. Peroneus longus tendon rupture as a cause of chronic lateral ankle pain. *Clin Orthop Relat Res.* 1999;(365):163-166.
77. Okazaki K, Nakashima S, Nomura S. Stress fracture of an os peroneum. *J Orthop Trauma.* 2003;17(9):654-656.

6

Posterior Tibial Tendon Pathology

Keith Wapner, MD

Introduction

Acute rupture of the posterior tibial tendon is very rare. It is often associated with medial malleolar fractures and can be identified by loss inversion and plantar flexion following trauma. Pain will be present along the posterior tibial tendon as well as the site of the medial malleolar fracture. X-rays will identify the fracture and magnetic resonance imaging (MRI) may be indicated to define the tendon pathology. The tendon should be surgically repaired at the time of operative treatment of the fracture.

Chronic degenerative tear of the posterior tibial tendon is the more common injury. This type of posterior tibial tendon

Hurwitz SR, Parekh SG. *Musculoskeletal Examination of the Foot and Ankle: Making the Complex Simple* (pp. 107-123). © 2012 SLACK Incorporated.

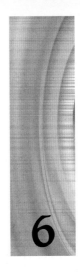

pathology has been identified as the most common cause of the adult acquired flat foot deformity.[1,2] The deterioration of the posterior tibial tendon leads to secondary collapse of the spring ligament. Although the exact etiology of chronic posterior tibial tendon dysfunction has not been identified, it has been associated with inflammatory, traumatic, and degenerative conditions.[3-6] It most commonly presents in the 50- to 60-year-old age group. Chronic posterior tibial tendinopathy presents as a continuum of deterioration, and the treatment protocol is dictated by the stage of deterioration identified at the time of the diagnosis.

History

Patients present without a history of an acute traumatic event. They describe a gradual onset of hindfoot pain with swelling along the medial aspect of the ankle.[7] Patients often note a progressive collapse of the medial longitudinal arch and will identify difficulty with activities that involve single heel raise such as going up and down the stairs or putting things up on a high shelf. They may also identify breakdown of the medial counter of the shoe and relate that the foot is collapsing while walking. As the symptoms worsen and the posterior tibial tendon goes onto complete rupture, the medial pain may diminish and the patient may present with lateral discomfort instead. This is caused by lateral impingement associated with progressive collapse of the medial longitudinal arch and loss of the spring ligament, causing impingement of the fibula onto the calcaneus and peroneal tendons.

In the early stages of the disease process, the patient may still be able to perform activities of daily living. As the tendon continues to deteriorate, the patient will present with more disability and increasing pain. In assessing these patients clinically, it is important to determine any previous treatment received prior to their presentation at your office.

Examination

Physical examination of the foot should include assessment of the standing posture of the foot as well as observation of the patient's gait. The patient should be observed from behind while standing. The position of the heel should be noted. There is generally increased valgus position of the calcaneus. In addition, the "too many toes" sign will be observed secondary to the collapse of the medial longitudinal arch and increased abduction of the foot. The reverse Coleman block test should be performed to determine if there is flexibility of the hindfoot.

The patient should also be asked to perform a single heel raise. Patients often have difficulty maintaining their balance when doing this. The patient should be instructed to hold on to the table for balance only, and then stand on the affected foot while raising the nonaffected foot by flexing the knee. The patient should then be asked to single heel raise on the affected foot without flexing his or her knee and without pushing off of the table.

The patient should also be examined in a seated position. While facing the patient, the foot should be held in a neutral posture and the forefoot should be assessed. This allows differentiation between a fixed and flexible deformity. If the patient's heel is brought into a neutral posture and the forefoot is reducible to a neutral position, then the deformity is flexible. If the patient's forefoot cannot be reduced when the heel is in neutral, it would be consistent with a fixed deformity. The patient should then be asked to plantarflex and invert the foot against resistance. It is critical to keep the foot in maximum plantar flexion while the foot inverts to isolate the posterior tibial tendon. The strength of the tendon can be assessed by pushing the forefoot into an adducted plantar flexed position against your hand. At the same time, palpating along the posterior tibial tendon can identify bogginess and thickening of the tendon as well as tenderness within the tendon sheath itself. The heel should then be reduced to neutral and the forefoot should be reduced to a neutral posture by manipulating the midfoot to make sure that the talar head is covered by the navicular. With the foot in this position, dorsiflexion of the foot should be tested with the knee both in a fully extended as well as a flexed position to assess combined gastroc-soleus or isolated gastroc tightness.

PATHOANATOMY

The posterior tibial tendon arises from the posterior tibial muscle just proximal to the medial malleolus and continues within its sheath behind the posterior aspect of the medial malleolus extending down to its insertions on the navicular and cuneiforms. The mesotenon blood supply of the tendon terminates 1 cm distal to the medial malleolus and the distal blood supply comes from the periosteal vessels near the insertion, leaving a hypovascularized area of the tendon between these 2 areas. This is the most common area to see the development of posterior tibial tendon pathology. As the posterior tibial tendon continues to deteriorate, increasing stress is placed on the spring ligament. This often leads to secondary deterioration of the spring ligament, which increases the abduction of the forefoot and collapse of the medial longitudinal arch.[8]

With the loss of the posterior tibial tendon function, the transverse tarsal joints' abilities to adduct, invert, and plantarflex are lost, causing peritalar subluxation of the joints. The ability to perform single heel raise is diminished secondary to loss of the rigid lever that is produced by midfoot adduction and calcaneal inversion.

With progressive loss of the posterior tibial tendon function, the antagonistic force to the peroneus brevis is lost. The unopposed pull of the peroneus brevis increases the strain of the spring ligament and causes further abduction of the forefoot. The progressive loss of the medial longitudinal arch occurs from the combined loss of the function of the posterior tibial tendon, progressive attenuation, and loss of the spring ligament. This leads to further strain on the deltoid ligament and may lead to attenuation of the deltoid.

With progressive collapse of the medial stabilizing structures, the calcaneus progressively collapses into a more valgus position, allowing the talar head to plantarflex. This is worsened by the progressive adduction of the navicular off of the talar head. This causes loss of the normal calcaneal pitch, which can then lead to progressive heel cord contraction. The progressive collapse of the subtalar and transverse tarsal joints leads to progressive peritalar subluxation. This can ultimately lead to degenerative changes within the subtalar and transverse tarsal joint complex, causing progressive rigidity of the deformity. This results in progressive loss of the deltoid

Table 6-1

STAGES OF POSTERIOR TIBIAL TENDON DYSFUNCTION

Stage I	Painful swollen posterior tibial tendon with minimal deformity
Stage II	Painful, swollen, thickened posterior tibial tendon with flexible pes planus deformity
Stage III	Painful, swollen, thickened, or absent posterior tibial tendon with fixed pes planus deformity
Stage IV	Painful, swollen, thickened, or absent posterior tibial tendon with fixed pes planus deformity and valgus ankle deformity

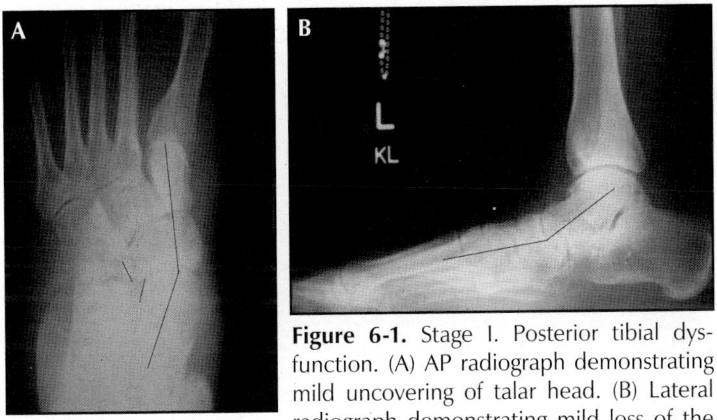

Figure 6-1. Stage I. Posterior tibial dysfunction. (A) AP radiograph demonstrating mild uncovering of talar head. (B) Lateral radiograph demonstrating mild loss of the normal talonavicular angle.

ligament, leading to secondary talar tilt and ankle arthritis. In the end stages of this deformity, because of the increasing valgus of the calcaneus, there can be direct contact between the distal fibula and lateral wall of the calcaneus with increasing lateral impingement pain and subluxation or degenerative tearing of the peroneal tendons.

Posterior tibial tendon dysfunction presents as a continuum of progressive deformity and has been classified into stages of disease (Table 6-1).[1,2,9] Stage I presents with inflammation within the tendon sheath with minimal damage to the tendon but no significant lengthening (Figure 6-1). Stage II presents with progressive disruption of the posterior tibial tendon

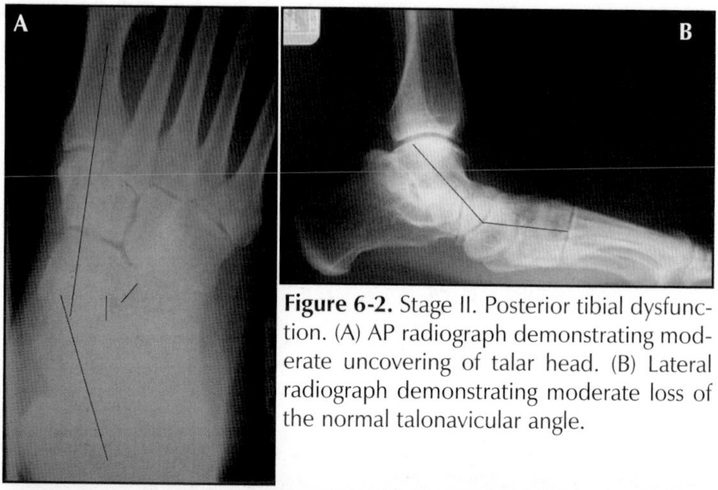

Figure 6-2. Stage II. Posterior tibial dysfunction. (A) AP radiograph demonstrating moderate uncovering of talar head. (B) Lateral radiograph demonstrating moderate loss of the normal talonavicular angle.

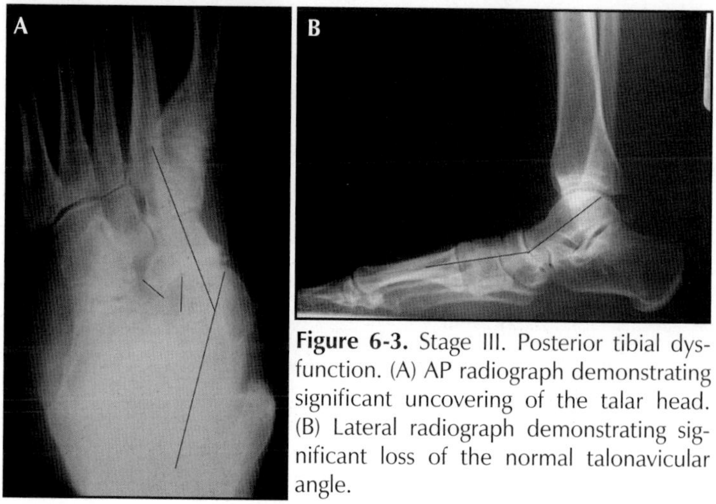

Figure 6-3. Stage III. Posterior tibial dysfunction. (A) AP radiograph demonstrating significant uncovering of the talar head. (B) Lateral radiograph demonstrating significant loss of the normal talonavicular angle.

with increasing calcaneal valgus and abduction of the forefoot (Figure 6-2). Stage III presents with significant calcaneal valgus and forefoot abduction and becomes rigid (Figure 6-3). Stage IV is defined as a Stage III deformity with secondary degenerative changes involving the ankle joint (Figure 6-4). The treatment protocols are dependent upon the assessment of the degree of tearing of the tendon and secondary bony changes and the flexibility or rigidity of the foot (Table 6-2).

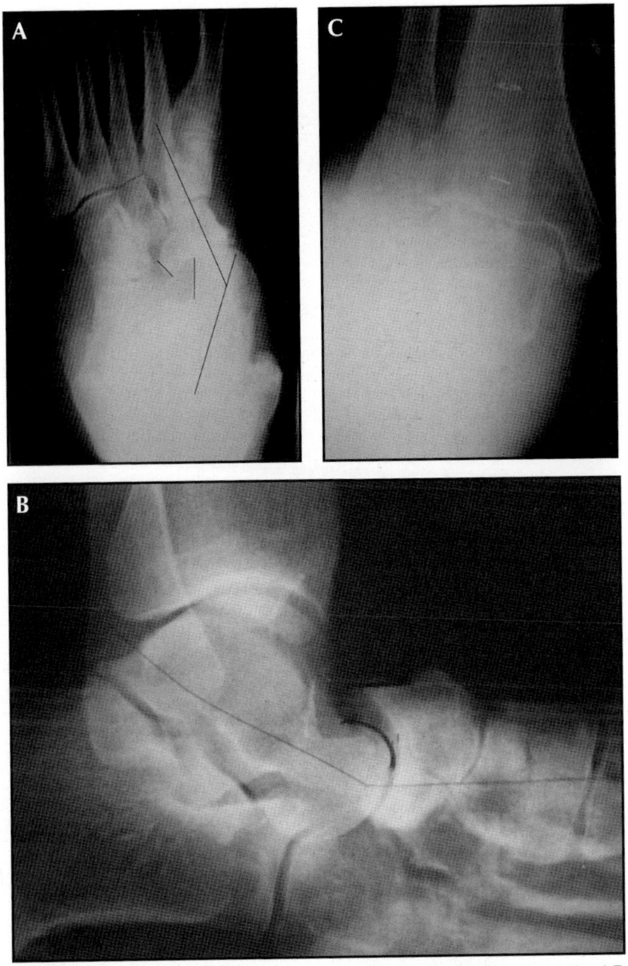

Figure 6-4. Stage IV. Posterior tibial dysfunction. (A) AP radiograph demonstrating severe uncovering of talar head. (B) Lateral radiograph demonstrating severe loss of the normal talonavicular angle. (C) AP ankle radiograph demonstrating valgus malalignment of the ankle secondary to compromise of the deltoid ligament.

Table 6-2

Methods for Examination

Examination	*Technique*	*Illustration*	*Grading/Characteristics*	*Significance*
Muscle testing	Plantarflex ankle and invert subtalar joint against resistance	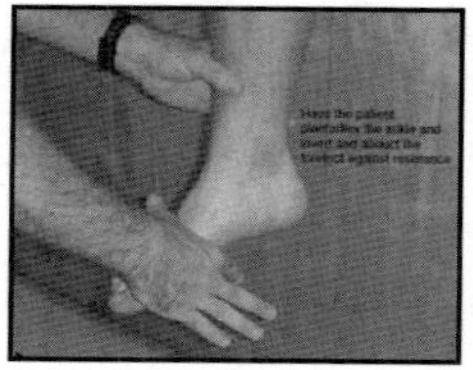	Muscle strength may be evaluated in 5 grades (0 to 5, Oxford scale) 0 = No muscle activity 1 = Muscle contraction; no movement 2 = Able to move in direction of gravity 3 = Movement against gravity 4 = Movement against resistance 5 = Movement against full resistance	Decreased strength indicates tendinosis Absent strength indicates complete tear
"Too many toes" sign	Observe patient from behind and compare with other foot	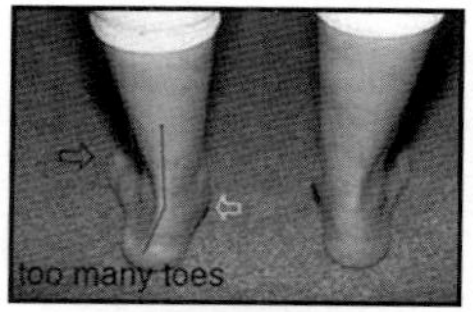	Cannot single heel raise, forefoot stays abducted and heel remains in valgus More toes visualized than nonaffected foot	"Too many toes" sign indicates elongation of posterior tibial tendon and spring ligament
Single heel raise	Stand on affected leg and try to raise onto forefoot	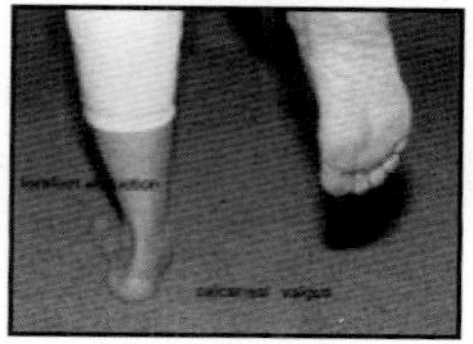	Can single heel raise with calcaneus going into varus Can single heel raise with difficulty and pain with calcaneus going into neutral or varus Cannot single heel raise, forefoot stays abducted and heel remains in valgus	Tendinosis but intact Tendinosis with partial tear Complete tear

Imaging

Standing AP, lateral, and oblique x-rays of the foot as well as standing AP, lateral, and mortise views of the ankle are used. The ankle x-rays are important in assessing the position of the talus within the ankle mortise. In the later stages of the disease, loss of deltoid function can lead to a valgus deformity of the talus within the ankle mortise, causing lateral impingement and degenerative arthritis of the ankle. AP, lateral, and oblique x-rays of the foot are important for assessing the calcaneal pitch as well as the alignment of the talonavicular and navicular cuneiform first metatarsal. With progressive deformity, there is progressive loss of the normal calcaneal pitch and progressive sag at the level of the talonavicular joint. In addition, increased medial stress may lead to plantar gapping of the first metatarsocuneiform or navicular medial cuneiform articulation. Assessment of the AP radiographs identifies the proper alignment of the navicular over the talar head. Progressive lateral deviation of the navicular secondary to the abduction of the forefoot can be identified (see Figure 6-3A). The presence and absence of degenerative changes should be noted.

MRI scans are helpful in defining the degree of tendon dysfunction.[10] The MRI classifications are based on the degree of tearing and hypertrophy of the tendon but do not directly correlate to the clinical staging. Type I demonstrates a partial tear of the tendon with hypertrophy and heterogeneous signal intensities with linear or round areas of increased signal. Type II demonstrates more severe partial tearing and thinning or attenuation of the tendon. There may be hypertrophy proximal and distal to the attenuated segment. Type III demonstrates a complete tear of the tendon with fluid in the tendon sheath.

Ultrasound can also be used to identify posterior tibial tendon pathology.[11] It has the advantage of being a less expensive study but is more operator dependent than MRI imaging. In general, orthopedic surgeons are more familiar with reviewing the MRI imaging than ultrasound imaging.

Treatment

Treatment of posterior tibial tendon dysfunction is guided by the clinical stage of deformity (Table 6-3). Both the extent of damage to the tendon, secondary changes of the ankle, subtalar, transverse tarsal, and first metatarsocuneiform joints need to be assessed. The condition of the spring ligament should be considered as well. In addressing the patients with posterior tibial tendon insufficiency, proximal deformity in the knee should also be evaluated. The patient should be presented with the surgical and nonsurgical options for treatment. Nonsurgical treatment may be successful in resolving Stage I and early Stage II deformities. Nonsurgical options with bracing can provide long-term pain relief in the later stages of posterior tibial tendon dysfunction but are unsuccessful in restoring normal function to the tendon.

Stage I posterior tibial tendon dysfunction can often be managed without surgical treatment. When the patient is diagnosed, his or her ankle and foot should be immobilized with an ankle-foot orthosis (Figure 6-5). This period of immobilization should be followed by appropriate rehabilitation. Because the immobilization often extends beyond 1 or 2 months, many physicians will utilize a nonarticulating polypropylene ankle-foot orthosis or an Arizona (ArizonaAFO, Mesa, AZ) or South West (South West Orthopedic Designs, LLC, Phoenix, AZ) type brace to allow the patients to undergo immobilization without the need for a more cumbersome cast or cast walker.[12] The immobilization can be accompanied by a nonsteroidal anti-inflammatory drugs (NSAIDs). Once the inflammation of the tendon begins to diminish, the patient can begin active range of motion exercises to prevent stenosis of the tendon. As the patient is able to tolerate active range of motion without pain, the patient can progress to strengthening exercises and then gradually wean off of the brace.[13] If the immobilization is not successful in resolving the inflammatory tenosynovitis of the tendon after a period of 3 to 6 months, operative tenosynovectomy can be considered followed by a rehabilitation program.

The treatment of Stage II posterior tibial tendinosis is dependent on multiple factors. Conservative management with bracing can be utilized for pain control but is less likely to result in

Table 6-3

Helpful Hints

Stage	*Radiology*	*Treatment*
Stage I		
Swollen tendon No deformity	X-ray: Normal alignment MRI: Synovitis of sheath Thickened tendon	Brace NSAID Physical therapy
Stage II		
Swollen tendon Calcaneal valgus Forefoot abduction Flexible	X-ray: Mild peritalar subluxation MRI: Synovitis of sheath; thickened tendon; increased signal in the tendon	Brace Flexor digitorum longus (FDL) transfer Medial displacement calcaneal osteotomy Lateral column lengthening
Stage III		
Swollen tendon Calcaneal valgus Forefoot abduction Rigid	X-ray: Increased peritalar subluxation MRI: Synovitis of sheath; thickened tendon; increased signal in the tendon or torn tendon	Brace Triple arthrodesis
Stage IV		
Swollen tendon Calcaneal valgus Forefoot abduction Rigid or flexible Ankle deformity	X-ray: Increased peritalar subluxation Ankle arthritis and valgus malalignment MRI: Synovitis of sheath; thickened tendon; increased signal in the tendon or torn tendon	Brace Pantalar fusion Triple arthrodesis with deltoid reconstruction

restoration of normal function of the tendon. In patients that are nonoperative candidates or do not wish to undergo surgery, similar bracing techniques as used with Stage I are often effective in controlling their discomfort.

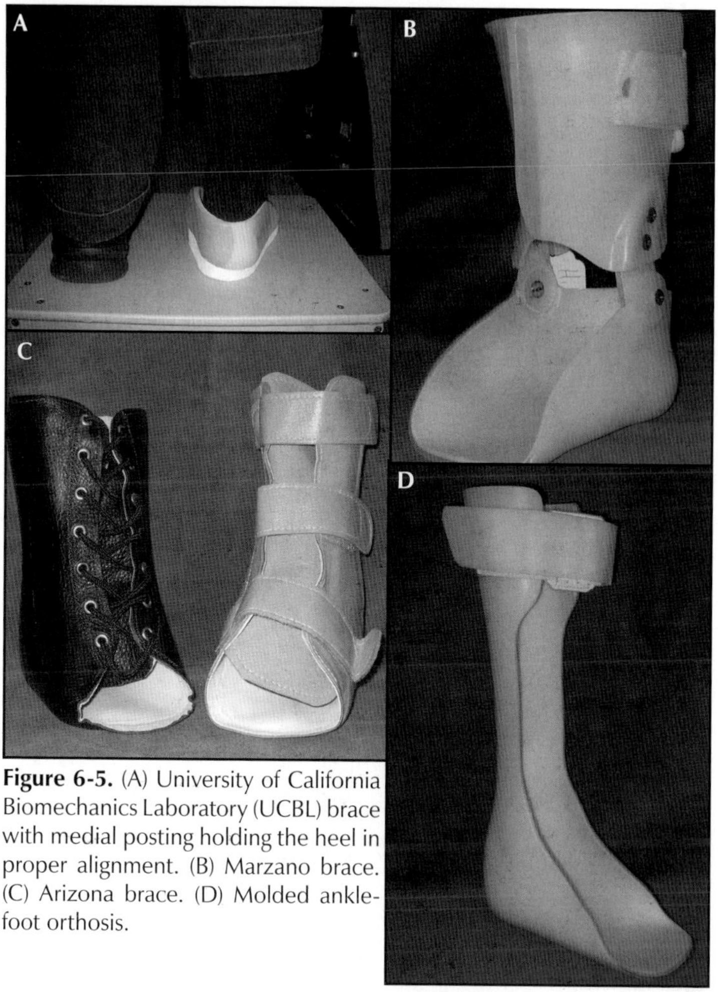

Figure 6-5. (A) University of California Biomechanics Laboratory (UCBL) brace with medial posting holding the heel in proper alignment. (B) Marzano brace. (C) Arizona brace. (D) Molded ankle-foot orthosis.

Operative treatment of the tendon dysfunction is most commonly achieved with débridement or excision of the diseased portion of the posterior tibial tendon and transfer of the FDL tendon into the posterior tibial tendon sheath (Figure 6-6). The tendon is then placed through a drill hole in the navicular to mimic the anatomic insertion of the posterior tibial tendon insertion. The condition of the spring ligament should be assessed at the time of surgery (Figure 6-7), and if that ligament is torn, it should be repaired.[14]

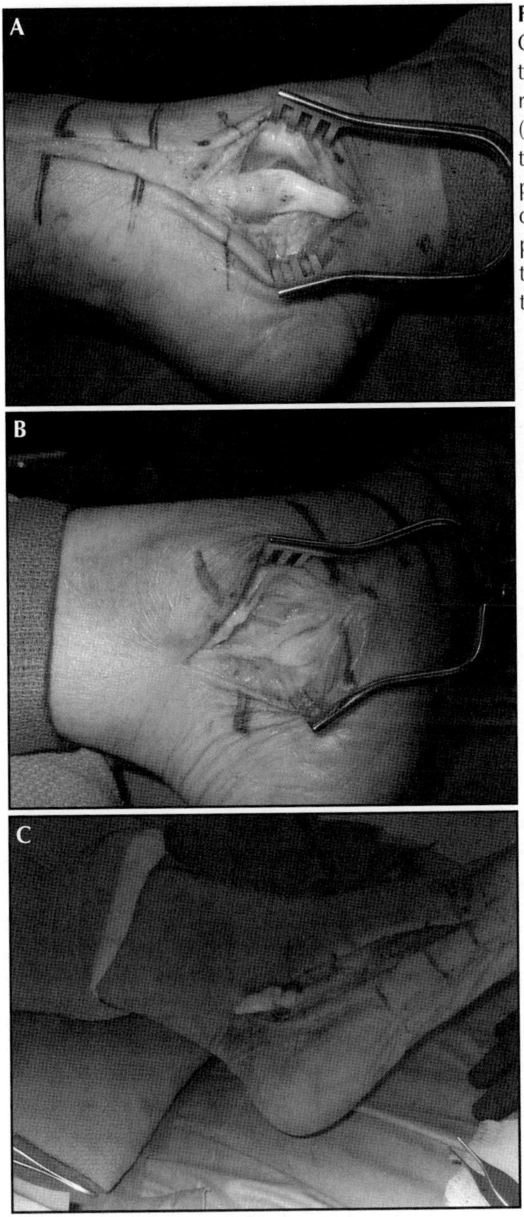

Figure 6-6. (A) Complete distal tear of the posterior tibial tendon. (B) Multiple longitudinal tears of the posterior tibial tendon. (C) Complete proximal tear of the posterior tibial tendon.

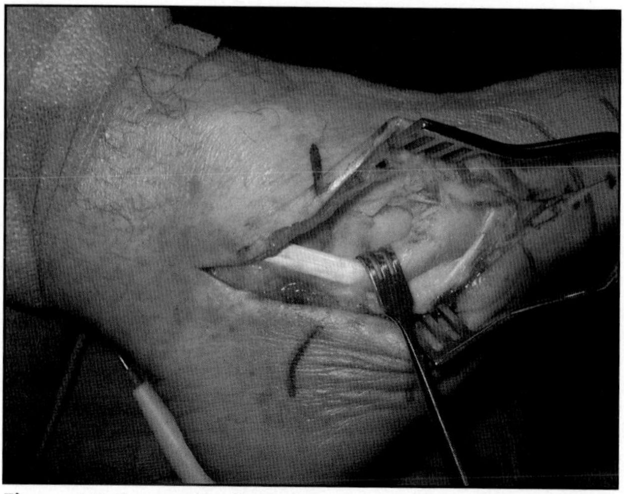

Figure 6-7. Torn spring ligament.

If there is a fixed contracture of the heel cord, then a tendon Achilles lengthening or gastroc-soleus lengthening with Strayer procedure can be considered. Concomitant bony procedures are often utilized and this is determined by the degree of peritalar subluxation. The indications for these bony procedures remain controversial. If there is isolated calcaneal valgus with minimal forefoot abduction, then a medial displacement calcaneal osteotomy is often utilized.[15,16] The medial displacement of the calcaneus medializes the force of the Achilles tendon and allows it to assist in the function of the posterior tibial tendon (Figure 6-8).

If there is significant forefoot adduction then consideration of a lateral column lengthening through the calcaneus can be employed. By lengthening the calcaneus, this will help to medialize the navicular to restore more normal coverage of the talar head.[17] Various techniques of achieving this lateral column lengthening have been employed (Figure 6-9). If there is associated instability of the first ray with gapping at the first metatarsocuneiform joint, either an open wedge first cuneiform osteotomy can be employed or a fusion of the first metatarsocuneiform joint can be utilized. The FDL tendon transfer and the various osteotomies are indicated in flexible deformities in the absence of degenerative arthritis.

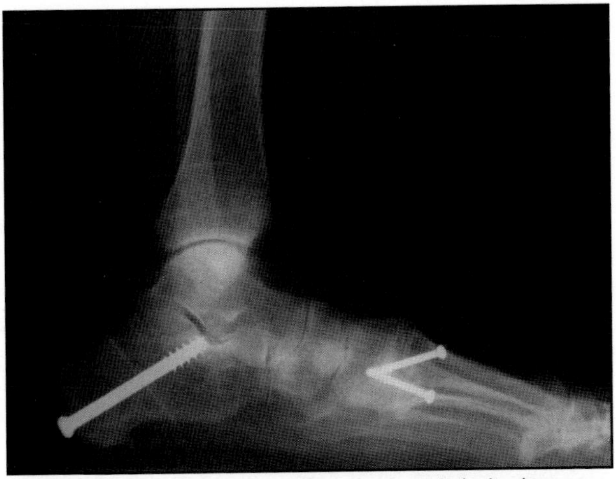

Figure 6-8. Lateral radiograph after medial displacement calcaneal osteotomy.

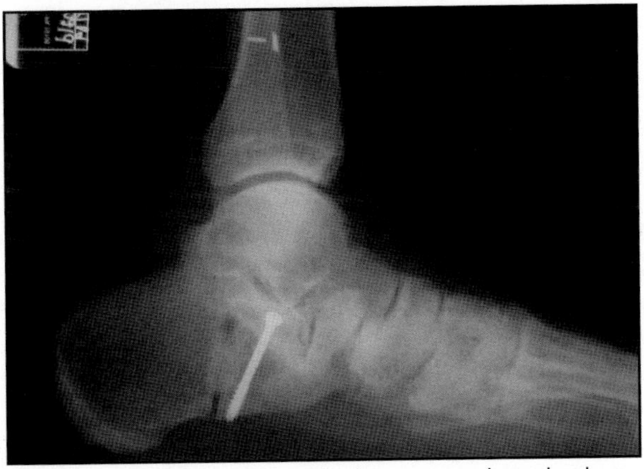

Figure 6-9. Lateral radiograph after step cut lateral column lengthening calcaneal osteotomy.

In Stage III posterior tibial tendon dysfunction where there is a rigid deformity and the presence of the arthritis, a triple arthrodesis with realignment of the subtalar and transverse tarsal and talonavicular joints into an anatomic position is generally employed.

In Stage IV, posterior tibial tendon dysfunction is less well defined. If there is a rigid hindfoot, it can be addressed by performing a triple arthrodesis. It is essential to restore a plantigrade position of the foot to decrease the stress on the ankle joint. If there is an ankle deformity without significant arthritis, reconstruction of the deltoid ligament can be attempted. If there are degenerative changes of the ankle joint, then a pantalar fusion may be required. If the integrity of the deltoid ligament can be restored and a plantigrade foot can be achieved through a triple arthrodesis, consideration of treating the ankle arthritis with ankle replacement may be entertained.

In the patient who is not a good operative candidate, bracing can always be entertained. In general, in Stage II and Stage III the use of an Arizona or Southwest type brace may be adequate to control the patient's symptoms. In Stage IV with concomitant ankle arthropathy in patients that are significantly overweight, a longer lever arm is often required and the use of a molded ankle-foot orthosis may be required.

Conclusion

Posterior tibial tendon dysfunction is a continuum of disease. The appropriate treatment is based on recognizing the stage of tendon pathology when the patient presents to the office. Both nonoperative and operative options can be employed. The goals of treatment are pain relief and restoration of function. In the early stages of posterior tibial pathology without the presence of arthritis or rigid deformities, normal function of the foot can be restored. In the later stages of disease, the stability is generally achieved through arthrodesis and pain relief is generally accomplished but normal restoration of the foot function is not possible.

References

1. Johnson KA, Strom DE. Tibialis posterior tendon dysfunction. *Clin Orthop Relat Res*. 1989;(239):196-206.
2. Myerson MS, Badekas A, Schon LC. Treatment of stage II posterior tibial tendon deficiency with flexor digitorum longus tendon transfer and calcaneal osteotomy. *Foot Ankle Int*. 2004;25(7):445-450.

3. Holmes GB, Mann RA. Possible epidemiological factors associated with rupture of the posterior tibial tendon *Foot Ankle.* 1992;13(2):70-79.
4. Jahss MH. Spontaneous rupture of the tibialis posterior tendon: clinical findings, tenographic studies, and a new technique repair. *Foot Ankle.* 1982;3(3):158-166.
5. Mosier SM, Luca DR, Pomeroy G, Manoli A II. Pathology of the posterior tibial tendon in the posterior tibial tendon insufficiency. *Foot Ankle Int.* 1998;19(8):520-524.
6. Rosenberg ZS, Cheung Y, Jahss MH, Noto AM, Norman A, Leeds NE. Rupture of posterior tibial tendon: CT and MR imaging with surgical correlation. *Radiology.* 1988;169(1):229-235.
7. Mizel MS, Hecht, PH, Marymont JV, Temple HT. Evaluation and treatment of chronic ankle pain. *Instr Course Lect.* 2004;53:311-321.
8. Mizel MS, Temple HT, Scranton PE Jr, et al. Role of the peroneal tendons in the production of the deformed foot with posterior tibial deficiency. *Foot Ankle Int.* 1999;20(5):285-289.
9. Bluman EM, Title CI, Myerson MS. Posterior tibial tendon rupture: a refined classification system. *Foot Ankle Clin.* 2007;12(2):233-249, v.
10. Sammarco GJ, Hockenbury RT. Treatment of stage II posterior tibial tendon dysfunction with flexor hallucis longus tendon transfer and medial displacement calcaneal osteotomy. *Foot Ankle Int.* 2001;22(4):305-312.
11. Miller SD, Marnix VH, Boruta PM Wu KK, Katcherian DA. Ultrasound in the diagnosis of posterior tibial tendon pathology. *Foot Ankle Int.* 1996;17(9):555-558.
12. Augustin JF, Lin SS, Berberian WS, Johnson JE. Nonoperative treatment of adult acquired flat foot with the Arizona brace. *Foot Ankle Clin.* 2003; 8(3):491-502.
13. Alvarez RG, Marini A, Schmitt C, Saltzman CL. Stage I and II posterior tibial tendon dysfunction treated by a structured nonoperative protocol: an orthosis and exercise program. *Foot Ankle Int.* 2006; 27(1):2-8.
14. Gazdag AR, Cracchiolo A III. Rupture of the posterior tibial tendon: Evaluation of injury of the spring ligament and clinical assessment of tendon transfer and ligament repair. *J Bone Joint Surg Am.* 1997;79(5):675-681.
15. Pinney SJ, Lin SS. Current concept review: acquired adult flatfoot deformity. *Foot Ankle Int.* 2006;27(1):66-75.
16. Wapner KL, Chao W. Nonoperative treatment of posterior tibial tendon dysfunction. *Clin Orthop Relat Res.* 1999;(365):39-45.
17. Dumontier TA, Falicov A, Mosca V, Sangeorzan B. Calcaneal lengthening: investigation of the deformity correction in a cadaver flatfoot model. *Foot Ankle Int.* 2005;26(2):166-170.

7

Pes Cavus

Lew Schon, MD and Adam T. Groth, MD

Introduction

The term *pes cavus* encompasses a spectrum of conditions defined by an abnormally high-arched foot. The primary factors for development of the pes cavus deformity are muscular imbalances stemming from neuromuscular, congenital, or traumatic disorders (Table 7-1). Varying definitions can be found depending on the etiology and whether the disease pattern primarily affects the hindfoot, the forefoot, or a combination of both. The degree of deformity can range from a mild cavus foot with flexible claw toes to a severe rigid deformity with altered weight bearing, plantar callosities, lateral ankle laxity, stress reactions, abnormal gait, and pain.[1] The goal

Hurwitz SR, Parekh SG. *Musculoskeletal Examination of the Foot and Ankle: Making the Complex Simple* (pp. 124-144).

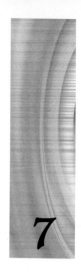

Table 7-1

Etiology of Pes Cavus

Neuromuscular	
Muscle disease	Muscular dystrophy
Afflictions of peripheral nerves and lumbosacral spinal nerve roots	Charcot-Marie-Tooth disease Spinal dysraphism Polyneuritis Traumatic peroneal palsy Intraspinal tumor
Disease of the anterior horn cell of the spinal cord	Poliomyelits Spinal dysraphism Diastematomyelia Syringomyelia Spinal cord tumors Spinomuscular atrophy
Long tract and central disease	Cerebral palsy Roussy-Lévy syndrome Primary cerebellar disease Friedreich's ataxia
Congenital	
	Idiopathic cavus foot Residual of clubfoot Arthrogryposis
Traumatic	
	Residual of compartment syndrome Crush injury Severe burns Fracture malunion Nerve laceration Tendon laceration

Adapted from Ibrahim K. Pes cavus. In: Evarts CM, ed. *Surgery of the Musculoskeletal System*. New York, NY: Churchill Livingstone; 1990:4015-4034.

in management of the cavus foot is to achieve a plantigrade painless stable foot and ankle with a smooth plantar pressure distribution.

History

Although the real incidence of cavus feet is currently unknown, a bell-shaped curve probably exists with high-arched cavus feet on one side and flatfeet on the other.[2] Some population-based studies suggest that the prevalence of pes cavus is approximately 10%.[3] The deformity rarely presents in young children but may develop as the child grows. Two-thirds of adults presenting with a symptomatic cavus foot have an underlying neuromuscular etiology arising from the central nervous system, spinal cord anomalies, or the peripheral nerves, most commonly Charcot-Marie-Tooth (CMT) disease.[4] Traumatic lesions must also be considered when evaluating muscular or structural problems of the foot as a pes cavus deformity may result from a compartment syndrome, nerve transection, crush injury, or tendon laceration. However, the largest single group is symmetric with no known etiology and the cause is labeled idiopathic.[1,5] The recognition of a rigid neuromuscular cavovarus foot may be readily apparent. Diagnosing the subtle cavus foot can be more challenging. A thorough history and physical examination including a detailed neurological evaluation are critical in determining the correct diagnosis as the etiology may affect prognosis and outcome.

Presenting complaints in patients with pes cavus may be related to a variety of associated conditions (Table 7-2) These complaints may be related to stiffness of the hindfoot, stress fractures along the lateral column (fifth metatarsal or cuboid), or recurrent ankle instability.[1] Significant peroneal tendon pathology may occur in the form of recurrent dislocation or subluxation, tendinitis, splitting, or painful os peroneum syndrome. Excessive plantar flexion of the first metatarsal and lateral column overload may lead to complaints of painful callosities (Figure 7-1), metatarsalgia, and hallux sesamoiditis. The abnormal mechanics of a stiff cavus foot may also lead to more proximal complaints, including stress fractures of

Table 7-2

CONDITIONS ASSOCIATED WITH THE CAVUS FOOT

Lateral ankle instability

Subtalar instability

Peroneal tendon pathology

- Peroneus brevis or longus tendon split
- Peroneal tendon dislocation or subluxation
- Enlarged peroneal tubercle
- Painful os peroneum syndrome

Stress fractures

- Base of the fourth or fifth metatarsal
- Cuboid
- Medial malleolus (vertical)
- Lateral malleolus
- Shin splints

Exertional compartment syndrome of leg, foot

Tight gastrocnemius muscle

Painful callosities at first and fifth metatarsal heads

Sesamoidal overload, chondromalacia, avascular necrosis

Plantar fasciitis

Metatarsus adductus

Arthritis

- Midfoot arthritis
- Subtalar arthritis
- Varus ankle arthritis
- Medial compartment knee arthritis

Iliotibial band friction syndrome

Adapted from Manoli A 2nd, Graham B. The subtle cavus foot, "the underpronator." *Foot Ankle Int.* 2005;26(3):256-263.

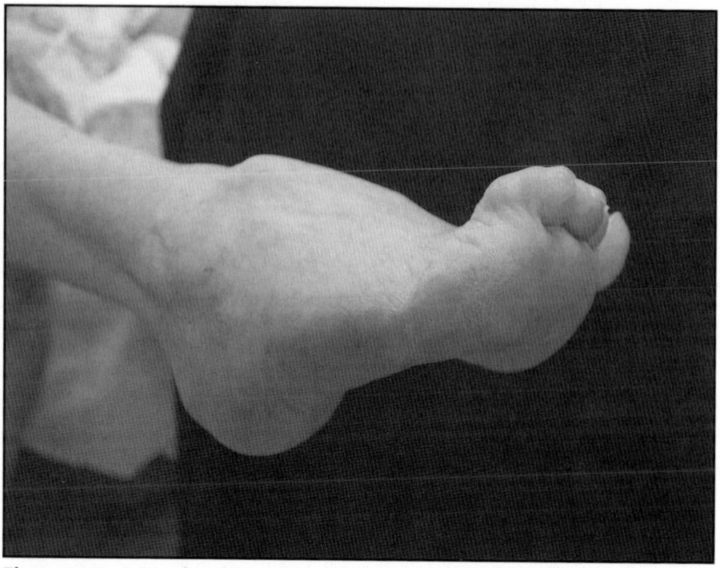

Figure 7-1. Lateral column overload with plantar callosities in patient with CMT.

the medial malleolus or fibula, shin splints, and exertional compartment syndrome.[2] Excessive external rotation of the talus and varus talar tilt may result in pain due to varus ankle arthritis, varus knee strain, and iliotibial band friction syndrome.[2] Patients may also provide a history of "underpronating" with increased lateral shoe wear (Figure 7-2).

Birth history, developmental delay, or family history of CMT, as well as hand, hip, foot, bowel, or bladder symptoms, should be noted.[6] Patients with CMT disease may also present with a history of fatigability manifesting as a dropfoot or steppage gait. A history of trauma in the form of a compartment syndrome, crush injury, severe burn, or fracture malunion (most commonly varus malunion of calcaneus or talar neck) may also cause a muscle imbalance leading to a cavus foot deformity.

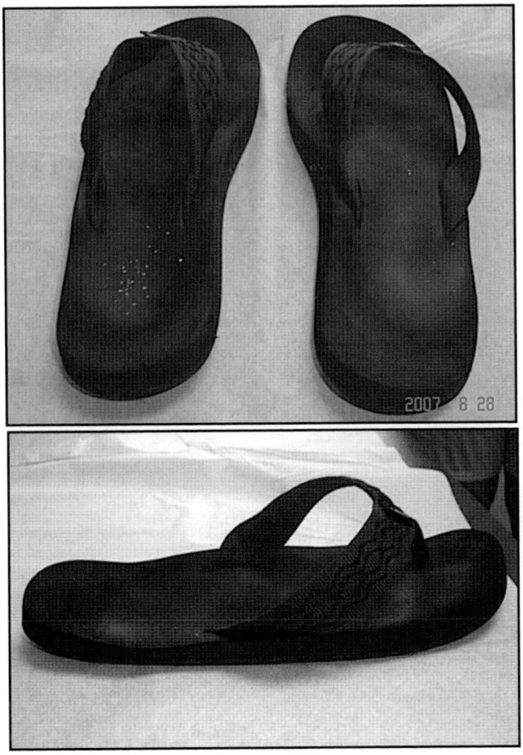

Figure 7-2. Lateral shoe wear in patient with idiopathic cavus foot.

Examination

The physical examination of the cavus foot is similar for other pathologic conditions of the foot and ankle, including inspection, palpation, range of motion testing, strength testing, and gait analysis (Table 7-3). The assessment should first begin with a standing inspection of the foot and evaluation of lower limb alignment. When viewing the normal foot from the front, the medial heel pad is not visible. With significant heel varus, a "peek-a-boo" heel sign occurs as the medial heel pad

Table 7-3

METHODS FOR EXAMINATION IN PES CAVUS

Examination	*Technique*	*Illustration*	*Grading and Significance*
Inspection	Foot alignment Claw toes Metatarsus adductus Forefoot pronation/plantar flexion of first ray	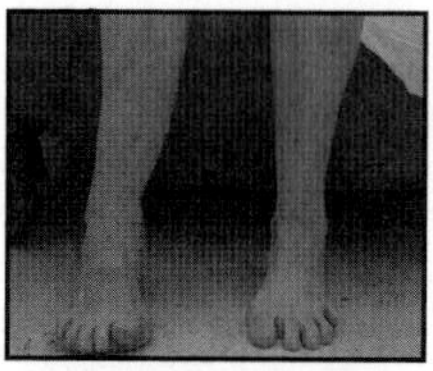	
	Limb alignment Ankle varus Tibia vara	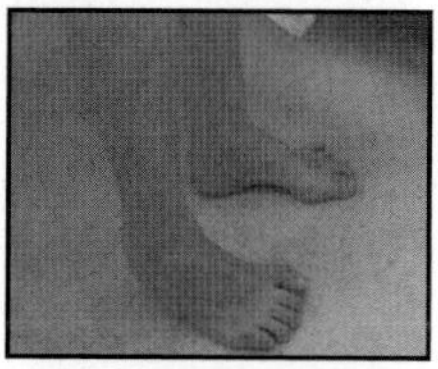	
	Plantar callosities/breakdown Shoe wear patterns	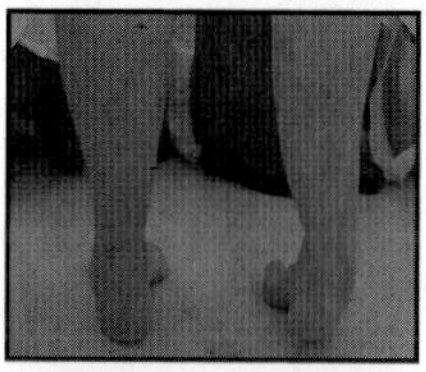	
Gait	1. Stance: Heel alignment Forefoot position	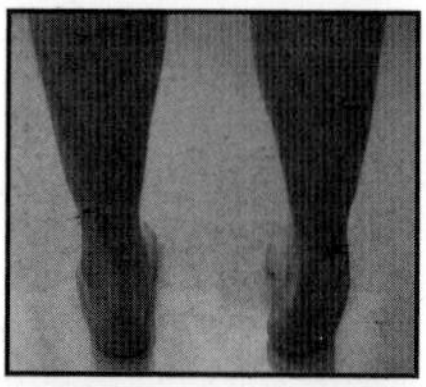	
	2. Swing: Foot drop/Steppage gait Cock up first MTP	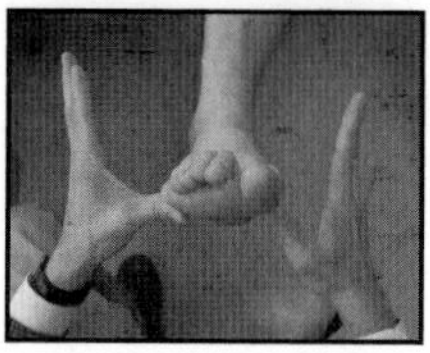	

(continued)

Table 7-3 (continued)

Methods for Examination in Pes Cavus

Examination	*Technique*	*Illustration*	*Grading and Significance*
Range of motion	Examine active and passive		
	1. Ankle		Normal: PF 50 degrees, DF 25 degrees
	2. Subtalar		Normal: Inv 25 to 30 degrees, Ever 5 to 10 degrees
	3. Transverse tarsal		Normal: Add 35 degrees, Abd 15 degrees
	4. Metatarso-phalangeal		Normal: PF 20 degrees, DF 60 degrees
Strength	Manual strength testing 1. Tibialis anterior 2. Extensor hallucis longus 3. Gastroc-soleus 4. Posterior tibialis 5. Flexor hallucis longus 6. Peroneus longus 7. Peroneus brevis 8. Hand intrinsics	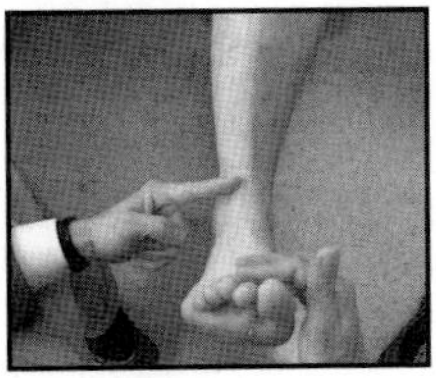	Grade 5 = Full strength Grade 4 = <Full strength Grade 3 = Movement with gravity Grade 2 = Movement without gravity Grade 1 = Visible contraction (Varying patterns of weakness or spasticity will determine deformity and treatment.)

(continued)

PF = plantar flexion; DF = dorsiflexion; Add = Addution; Abd = Abduction

Table 7-3 (continued)

Methods for Examination in Pes Cavus

Examination	*Technique*	*Illustration*	*Grading and Significance*
Neurologic	Sensation Deep tendon reflexes Upper motor neuron signs Vibratory Intrinsic wasting		Neurologic abnormality may be suggestive of a spinal cord lesion and mandates an MRI and neurology consultation
Coleman block test		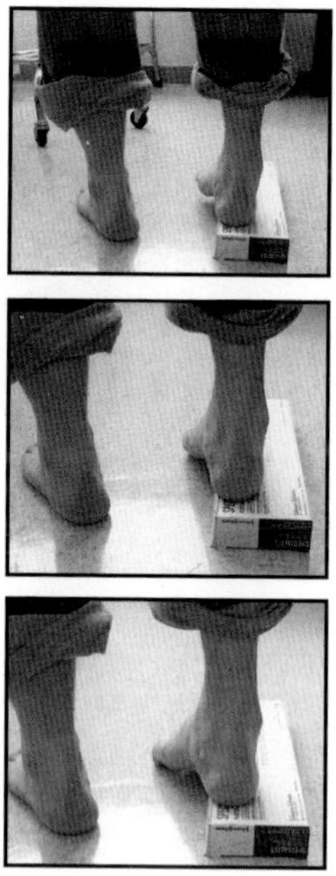	Determine the flexibility of the hindfoot and whether the deformity is driven more by the forefoot or hindfoot

(continued)

Table 7-3 (continued)

Methods for Examination in Pes Cavus

Examination	*Technique*	*Illustration*	*Grading and Significance*
Silfverskiold test	Evaluate ankle dorsiflexion at 0 degrees and 90 degrees of knee flexion	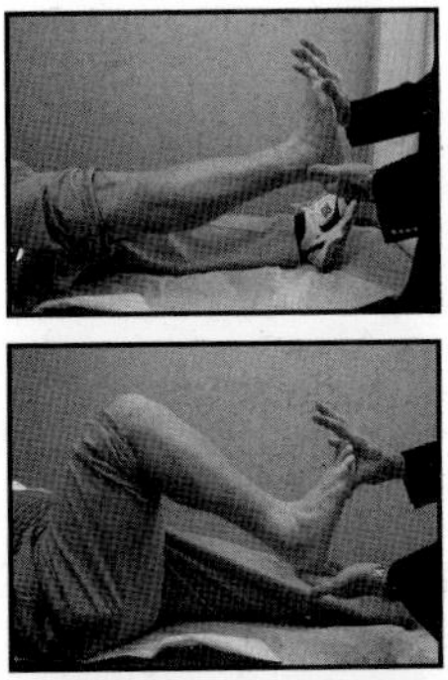	Achilles tendon lengthening or gastrocnemius recession is often required.
Anterior drawer	Stabilize tibia and grasp heel with foot in 25 degrees of plantar flexion. Evaluate translation as examiner pulls foot anteriorly and allows to internally rotate	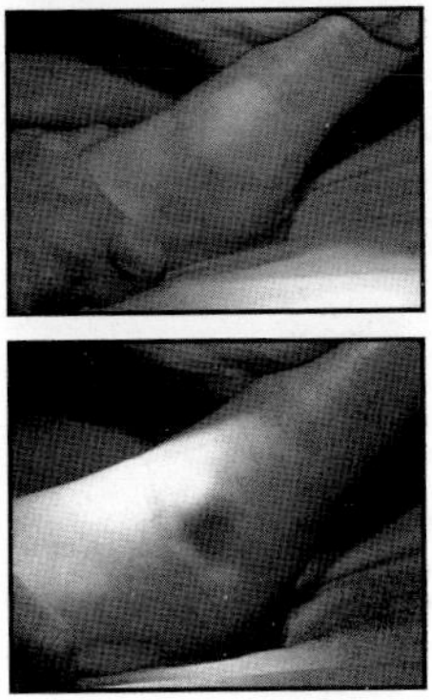	Indication of lateral ankle ligament instability. "Suction sign" may be visible over anterolateral corner of joint.

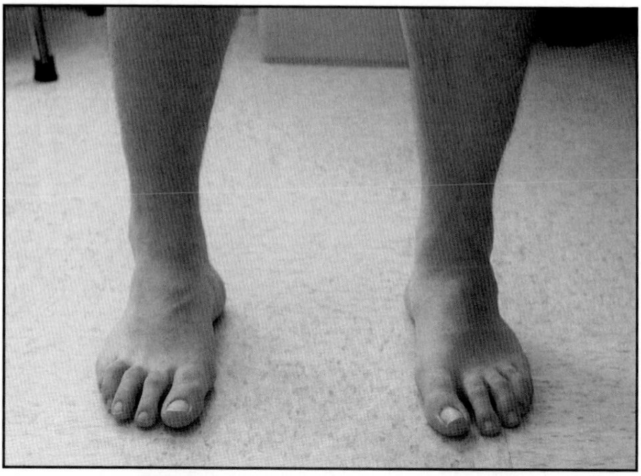

Figure 7-3. Peek-a-boo heel sign.

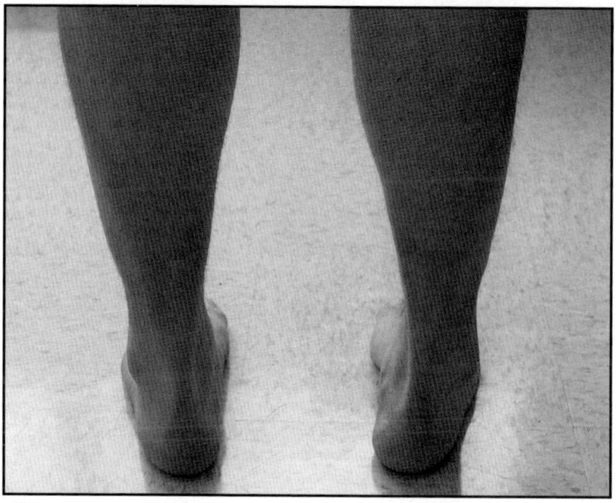

Figure 7-4. Hindfoot varus in patient with idiopathic cavus foot.

becomes apparent (Figure 7-3).[7] Metatarsus adductus, clawing of the toes, or any other forefoot abnormalities should be noted. When viewing the standing patient from behind, the calcaneus will be in varus in relation to the calf (Figure 7-4). Inspection of limb alignment should also note the presence of ankle varus (Figure 7-5), tibia vara, or any other alignment deformities. A Coleman block test will help determine the

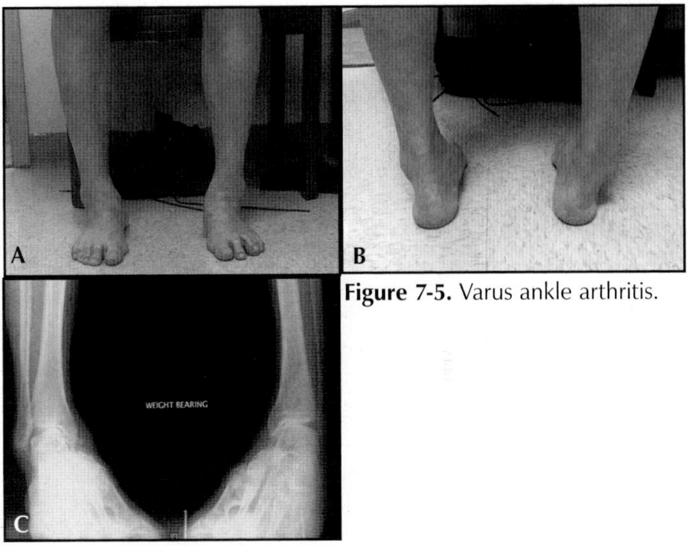

Figure 7-5. Varus ankle arthritis.

flexibility of the hindfoot and if the deformity is driven more by the forefoot or hindfoot. While observing the patient from behind, place a 1-in block under the heel and lateral forefoot, allowing the first 2 toes to fall into pronation off the medial edge of the block. If the hindfoot corrects to a normal valgus alignment, the cavus is forefoot driven and the hindfoot is flexible. If there is little or no correction with the block, the hindfoot is stiff in varus.[8]

Gait analysis should take into account the nature of ground contact, the position of the heel, and the position of the toes during stance. Some patients may demonstrate a greater progression of the heel toward hindfoot varus with weight bearing. A subtle foot drop may manifest as a steppage gait or cock up deformity of the first metatarsophalangeal joint during swing.

The remainder of the exam may be performed with the patient seated. Active and passive range of motion of the ankle, subtalar, transverse tarsal, and metatarsophalangeal joints should be noted. A stiff subtalar joint that is not correctable with the Coleman block test may also be indicative of a tarsal coalition or subtalar arthritis. The Silfverskiold test may be performed to evaluate gastrocnemius contracture. Forefoot

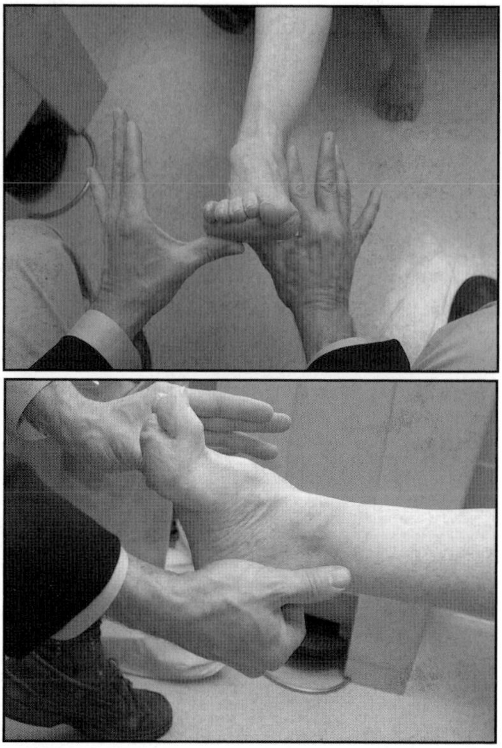

Figure 7-6. Forefoot varus with depression of first metatarsal head.

valgus is noted by depression of the first metatarsal head when looking at the cascade of the forefoot (Figure 7-6).

There may be variability in the pathomechanics that produce the different forms of cavus foot but all are related to muscle imbalance patterns. Specific attention must be given to evaluating the agonist-antagonist muscle relationships when testing motor strength. Resistance to depression of the first metatarsal head will test the strength of the peroneus longus (Figure 7-7A), while resistance to eversion of the lateral border of the foot will test peroneus brevis (Figure 7-7B).

Neurological testing should include screening for long tract signs, reflexes, and any asymmetry in motor pattern or deformity. Abnormality may be suggestive of a spinal cord lesion and mandates magnetic resonance imaging (MRI) and neurologic consultation. Intrinsic wasting of the hands and calf muscle atrophy may be observed in peripheral neuropathies such as CMT disease.

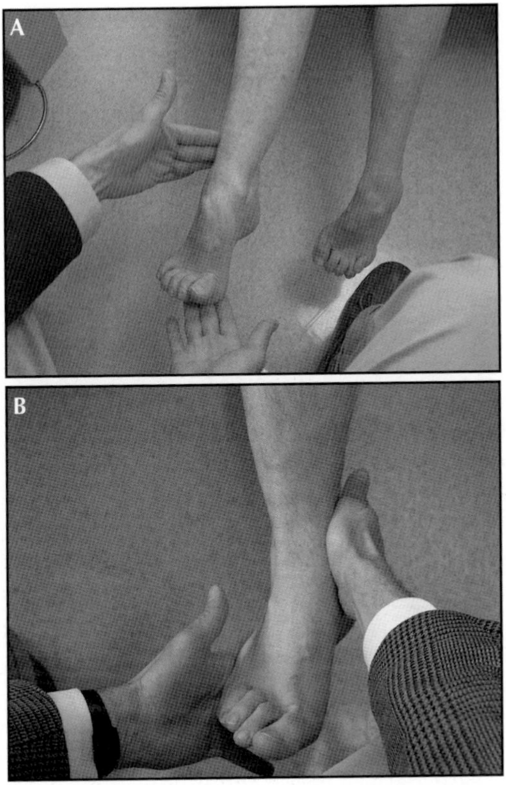

Figure 7-7. Strength testing of (A) peroneus longus and (B) peroneus brevis.

PATHOANATOMY

The cavus foot is best understood by systematically analyzing the bone deformities, soft tissue deformities, and specific muscle functions that are imbalanced. Hindfoot cavus refers to an elevated calcaneal pitch, usually greater than 30 degrees. Pure hindfoot cavus was traditionally seen as a result of poliomyelitis, but increased calcaneal pitch is now more commonly diagnosed as a component of a combined deformity in the idiopathic cavus foot.

Forefoot cavus describes plantar flexion of the metatarsals and is usually accompanied by forefoot adduction. The most common cause of pure forefoot cavus is CMT disease. It is critical to recognize that the forefoot cavus may cause the varus deformity of the hindfoot. Initially, the forefoot cavus is flexible and the subtalar joint falls into varus to compensate. As the disease progresses, the capsule and interosseous ligament of the subtalar joint become contracted and the flexible deformity becomes rigid. The metatarsophalangeal joint deformities are variable. Once rigid claw toe deformities develop, the forces of the extrinsic toe extensors hold the metatarsal heads in a plantarflexed position. In severe cases, the plantar fat pad displaces distally as the toes pull up into extension, leading to metatarsalgia. The plantar aponeurosis commonly becomes contracted. This structure is more stout medially, therefore as the contracture progresses, it not only holds the longitudinal arch in an elevated position, but it also holds the forefoot adducted and keeps the calcaneus inverted.[1]

The agonist-antagonist functional motor units of the lower extremity must be understood because varying patterns of weakness or spasticity will determine deformity and treatment. The posterior tibialis adducts the forefoot and inverts the hindfoot while the peroneus brevis everts it. The tibialis anterior dorsiflexes the first ray while the peroneus longus plantarflexes it. The triceps surae plantarflexes the foot while the tibialis anterior, extensor digitorum longus, and extensor hallucis longus work in opposition to it.

The foot deformities in CMT disease result from the selective denervation of muscles in the anterior and lateral compartments. The disease pattern most commonly affects the peroneus brevis and tibialis anterior muscles as well as the foot intrinsics but spares the peroneus longus and extensor hallucis longus. The unopposed posterior tibialis causes forefoot cavus with depression of the first metatarsal as well as supination and adduction of the forefoot. An equinus contracture results from the unopposed pull of the gastrocnemius. The unopposed toe extrinsics force the toes into a clawed position. The clawing of the hallux is worsened due to the unopposed action of the extensor hallucis longus.[9,10] The resultant deformity in poliomyelitis depends on what portion of the central nervous system is affected. With selective destruction of the anterior horn cells in the spinal cord and selective paralysis of the gastroc-soleus complex, a severe hindfoot cavus will occur. If the lesion is higher and affects the tibialis anterior, a forefoot cavus with clawing of the hallux occurs due to unopposed action of the peroneus longus and extensor hallucis longus.

Post-traumatic cavovarus foot deformities result from any condition that leads to an imbalance of the intrinsic and extrinsic musculature of the foot.

Adult clubfoot residual deformity may also present if initial attempts at serial casting did not adequately elevate the first ray prior to abducting the foot about the fulcrum of the talar head.[11] Placing the navicular in a dorsally subluxated position may also lead to a residual cavus deformity.[12]

Imaging

Standing anteroposterior (AP) and lateral radiographs of the feet are critical (Table 7-4). The lateral view (Figure 7-8) is helpful to define the apex of the deformity in the hindfoot, midfoot, or forefoot. Normal calcaneal pitch is 10 to 30 degrees and is measured between a line on the undersurface of the calcaneus and the floor. With hindfoot cavus there is increased dorsiflexion of the calcaneus and a calcaneal pitch >30 degrees. Hindfoot varus is noted as a "look through" sign over the posterior facet of the subtalar joint as there is no overlap of the lateral process of the calcaneus. The talar-first metatarsal angle, or Meary's angle, is formed between the long axes of the talus and the first metatarsal, and should be collinear. Plantar flexion of the first metatarsal is apparent in forefoot cavus. The AP radiograph (see Figure 7-8) should evaluate the presence of metatarsus adductus and metatarsal stress fractures. AP radiographs of the ankle should also be evaluated for talar tilt or ankle arthrosis (see Figure 7-5).

Further imaging modalities may be indicated to diagnose an associated condition. Unilateral or progressive cavus deformity or abnormal neurologic findings mandate further imaging of the spine with MRI. MRI of the lower extremity may show fatty infiltration in the peroneus brevis and anterior tibialis in CMT disease,[5] or enlargement of the peroneus longus in forefoot cavus.[13] Computed tomography (CT) scan may be helpful to rule out the presence of subtalar coalition. A bone scan may be used to diagnose stress reactions. Electromyographic studies and nerve conduction velocities may serve to diagnose a neuromuscular etiology.

Table 7-4

Helpful Hints

Imaging and Diagnostic Tests for the Cavus Foot

Weight-bearing plain radiograph (x-ray)	Lateral foot	Talar-first metatarsal angle (Normal: 0 degrees)
		Calcaneal pitch (Normal: 10 to 30 degrees)
		Subtalar "look through" sign
	AP foot	Metatarsus adductus
		Stress fractures
	AP ankle	Varus talar tilt
MRI		Peroneal tendon pathology
		Atrophy of muscle units
		Intraspinal lesions
CT scan		Subtalar coalition
Bone scan		Stress fractures
Electromyography		Neuropathy: Increased amplitude and duration of response
		Myopathy: Decreased amplitude and duration of response with short polyphasic potentials
		Denervation or anterior horn cell loss: Prolonged polyphasics, positive sharp waves, and fibrillations
Nerve conduction velociy (NCV)		Axonal degeneration: Prolonged latencies and minimal decrease in velocity

Treatment

The first step in management of the pes cavus deformity is the identification of a treatable underlying cause. The patient and family should be counseled about the natural history of

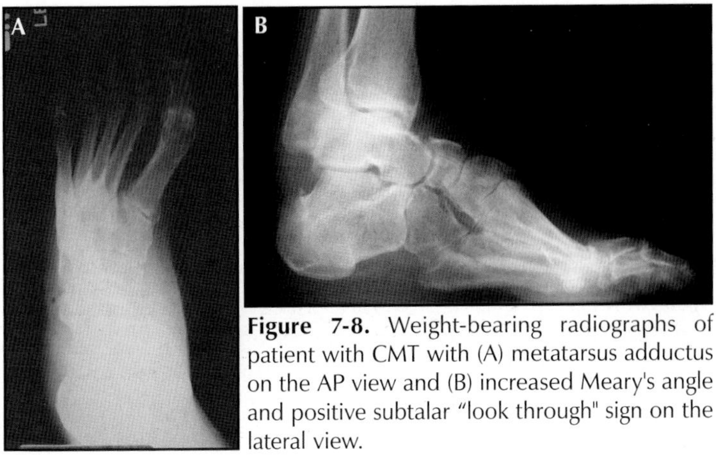

Figure 7-8. Weight-bearing radiographs of patient with CMT with (A) metatarsus adductus on the AP view and (B) increased Meary's angle and positive subtalar "look through" sign on the lateral view.

the deformity, and further neurologic and genetic workups should be pursued when indicated.

Nonoperative management may be appropriate for the patient with a mild or nonprogressive deformity. Conservative measures involve strategies to reduce and redistribute plantar pressure loading through the use of foot orthoses and specialized cushioned footwear,[14,15] which may include lateral forefoot posting, arch supports, and metatarsal bars. A recessed area for the first metatarsal head may allow the first metatarsal to further plantarflex and allow the hindfoot to evert to a more neutral position. Accommodative extra-depth shoes may be required in more advanced cases. Patients with significant weakness may require additional support in the form of an ankle-foot orthosis or double upright hinged orthosis. Other nonsurgical rehabilitation approaches include stretching and strengthening of tight and weak muscles (particularly the gastroc-soleus complex), débridement of plantar callosities, and strategies to improve balance.[2]

Surgery is indicated in cases refractory to conservative measures or situations in which an obvious muscle imbalance is expected to lead to progressive deformity. The procedures performed will depend on the age of the patient, the nature of the deformity, and the etiology. These procedures may be divided into soft tissue procedures, osteotomies, and arthrodesis procedures. Because the cavus foot may involve a spectrum of rigid and flexible deformities within each disease pattern, it may be necessary to utilize multiple procedures to address each deformity.

Soft tissue procedures include plantar fascia release, tendon lengthenings, and tendon transfers. Plantar fascia release may help reduce the height of the arch and is usually combined with other procedures in patients who have maintained some degree of flexibility. A subcutaneous plantar fascia release may be beneficial in isolation in young children with minimal fixed deformity.[16] Achilles tendon lengthening or gastrocnemius recession is required in most forefoot cavus corrections. A gastrocnemius contracture will potentiate a forefoot-driven cavus by increasing the relative strength of the peroneus longus as compared with the anterior tibialis.[2] The first toe Jones procedure is often used in CMT and variants of cerebral palsy to correct the cock up deformity of the first metatarsophalangeal joint due to a weak tibialis anterior. Transfer of the insertion of the extensor hallucis longus (EHL) to the first metatarsal neck allows the EHL to become an accessory ankle dorsiflexor and helps minimize depression of the first metatarsal. In the young patient with forefoot cavus and flexible hindfoot deformity due to overpull of the peroneus longus, a peroneus longus to brevis transfer may be helpful. Management of claw toe deformities depends upon whether they are fixed or flexible. Supple deformities may be managed with flexor-to-extensor transfers (Girdlestone-Taylor procedure), while fixed claw toes will require proximal interphalangeal joint (PIP) arthroplasty or arthrodesis.

When patients present with a fixed varus hindfoot deformity or fixed plantar flexion of the first ray but the remainder of the deformity is supple, correction may be achieved by augmenting the reconstruction with specific osteotomies. A rigid forefoot valgus deformity caused by plantar flexion of the first metatarsal can be treated with a dorsiflexion osteotomy of the first metatarsal base. A fixed varus deformity of the heel may be corrected with a Dwyer lateral closing wedge osteotomy.[17] If the patient has a severe calcaneal pitch with a calcaneocavus deformity, a Samilson crescentic osteotomy or a dorsal displacement sliding calcaneal osteotomy may be performed.

Various midfoot realignment osteotomies have been described for patients with forefoot equinus and the apex of the cavus deformity at the midtarsal joints. Depending on the nature of the deformity, the osteotomy can be performed with a uniplanar cut in which the distal segment is rotated and impacted as the forefoot is elevated, or a biplanar cut with a dorsally based wedge. These osteotomies may involve multiple intra-articular cuts and can lead to early arthrosis. Consideration should be given to performing an extra-articular osteotomy when possible, even though it may be distant to the true apex of the deformity.

More severe rigid deformities of the hindfoot may require triple arthrodesis to achieve correction. Additional procedures as previously described may still be required to augment the global correction. At times, standard techniques for joint preparation will not allow enough correction to achieve a plantigrade foot, therefore additional cuts may be required in the form of Siffert beak-type triple arthrodesis.[18] Though not contraindicated, it must be recognized that arthrodesis in this setting is associated with multiple complications, particularly ankle arthritis.

When addressing associated conditions such as lateral ankle instability, it is critical to recognize the contribution of the underlying foot alignment. If there is a fixed hindfoot varus deformity, the lateral ankle ligament reconstruction should be complemented by a Dwyer calcaneal osteotomy. If the hindfoot is more flexible and the varus is a result of a plantarflexed first ray, then the repair may be augmented by a dorsiflexion osteotomy of the first metatarsal. Pathologies associated with the cavus foot need to be corrected operatively as well as the structural components of the pes cavus deformity.[2]

Conclusion

The cavus foot is characterized by elevation of the medial longitudinal arch with varying degrees of medial forefoot plantar flexion and adduction and hindfoot varus. A thorough history and detailed physical examination are necessary to establish the proper diagnosis of a structural cavus foot deformity and the associated conditions that may accompany it. Understanding the etiology and recognizing the muscle imbalances causing the deformity are critical to establishing the proper treatment strategy.

References

1. Guyton GP, Mann RA. Pes cavus. In: Coughlin MJ, Mann RA, Saltzman CL, eds. *Surgery of the Foot and Ankle*. Philadelphia, PA: Mosby, Inc; 2007:1125-1148.
2. Manoli, A II, Graham B, The subtle cavus foot, "the underpronator". *Foot Ankle Int*. 2005;26(3):256-263.
3. Sachithanandam V, Joseph B. The influence of footwear on the prevalence of flat foot. A survey of 1846 skeletally mature persons. *J Bone Joint Surg Br*, 1995;77(2):254-257.
4. Alexander IJ, Johnson KA. Assessment and management of pes cavus in Charcot-Marie-Tooth disease. *Clin Orthop Relat Res*. 1989;(246):273-281.
5. Tynan MC, Klenerman L, Helliwell TR, Edwards RH, Hayward M. Investigation of muscle imbalance in the leg in symptomatic forefoot pes cavus: a multidisciplinary study. *Foot Ankle*. 1992;13(9):489-501.
6. Schwend RM, Drennan JC. Cavus foot deformity in children. *J Am Acad Orthop Surg*. 2003;11(3):201-211.
7. Beals TC, Manoli A II. The peak-a-boo heel sign in the evaluation of hindfoot varus. *Foot*. 1996;6:205-206.
8. Coleman SS. Chesnut WJ. A simple test for hindfoot flexibility in the cavovarus foot. *Clin Orthop Relat Res*. 1977;(123):60-62.
9. Guyton GP. Current concepts review: orthopaedic aspects of Charcot-Marie-Tooth disease. *Foot Ankle Int*. 2006;27(11):1003-1010.
10. Guyton GP, Mann RA. The pathogenesis and surgical management of foot deformity in Charcot-Marie-Tooth disease. *Foot Ankle Clin*. 2000;5(2):317-326.
11. Morcuende JA, Dolan LA, Dietz FR, Ponseti IV. Radical reduction in the rate of extensive corrective surgery for clubfoot using the Ponseti method. *Pediatrics*. 2004;113(2):376-380.
12. Simons GW. The complete subtalar release in club feet. Part II--Comparison with less extensive procedures. *J Bone Joint Surg Am* 1985;67(7):1056-1065.
13. Helliwell TR, Tynan M, Hayward M, Klenerman L, Whitehouse G, Edwards RH. The pathology of the lower leg muscles in pure forefoot pes cavus. *Acta Neuropathol*. 1995;89(6):552-559.
14. Burns J, Crosbie J, Ouvrier R, Hunt A. Effective orthotic therapy for the painful cavus foot: a randomized controlled trial. *J Am Podiatr Med Assoc*. 2006;96(3):205-211.
15. Crosbie J, Burns J. Predicting outcomes in the orthotic management of painful, idiopathic pes cavus. *Clin J Sport Med*. 2007;17(5):337-342.
16. Sherman FC, Westin GW. Plantar release in the correction of deformities of the foot in childhood. *J Bone Joint Surg Am*. 1981;63(9):1382-1389.
17. Dwyer FC. Osteotomy of the calcaneum for pes cavus. *J Bone Joint Surg Br*. 1959;41-B(1):80-86.
18. Siffert RS, Forster RI, Nachamie B. "Beak" triple arthrodesis for correction of severe cavus deformity. *Clin Orthop Relat Res*. 1966;45:101-106.

8

Achilles Pathology and Posterior Calcaneal Pain

Christopher P. Chiodo, MD and Antonio Gomez-Tristan, MD

Introduction

Patients with posterior heel and ankle pain are frequently encountered in both the general and subspecialized orthopedic practice. The physical examination and diagnostic approach to these patients should be anatomically based, and, as such, an understanding of the regional anatomy is essential.

The Achilles tendon, the strongest tendon of the human body, inserts onto the posterior tuberosity of the calcaneus. Disorders of the Achilles tendon are the most common cause of posterior heel pain. These include rupture, tendinosis, tendinitis, and bursitis. Acute Achilles ruptures have a reported incidence of approximately 18 per 100,000 people.[1,2] Tendinosis

Hurwitz SR, Parekh SG. *Musculoskeletal Examination of the Foot and Ankle: Making the Complex Simple* (pp. 145-156). © 2012 SLACK Incorporated.

Table 8-1

HELPFUL HINTS

Disorder	*Mechanism/Pathology*	*Presentation*
Achilles tendinosis/ tendinitis	Focal tendon degeneration/peritenon inflammation	Pain, tenderness, and nodularity at or above the Achilles insertion on the posterior calcaneal tuberosity
Retrocalcaneal bursitis	Bursal inflammation	Pain, tenderness, and fullness just anterior to the Achilles tendon
Achilles rupture	Acute injury, usually with eccentric contraction	"Pop" or "snap" in posterior ankle with acute weakness

and tendinitis, which can occur separately or together, are traditionally divided into insertional and noninsertional disease. Puddu and colleagues[3] further defined 3 distinct clinical entities: 1) peritendinitis, characterized by inflammation involving the peritendinous structures; 2) peritendinitis with tendinosis, in which there is also degeneration of the tendon itself; and 3) tendinosis, characterized by tendon degeneration without concomitant inflammation.

HISTORY

Patients who sustain an acute rupture of the Achilles tendon typically report a sudden "pop" or "snap" in the back of the ankle (Table 8-1). In some cases, this is actually audible. Athletes often think that they were struck, kicked, or hit by another player. While an acute Achilles rupture is accompanied by immediate pain and weakness, it is important to note that many patients are still able to walk. This may be responsible for the fact that up to 25% of these injuries may initially go unrecognized.[4,5]

Meanwhile, patients with Achilles tendinosis or tendinitis give a history of chronic posterior ankle and hindfoot pain. While the pain may vary in nature (eg, sharp, aching, dull), it often radiates up the posterior leg. It may also be worse in the morning or when first getting up after sitting for a long period of time. It is exacerbated by walking uphill and athletic activity, especially sports that entail jumping and high impact. Patients may complain of thickening and nodularity in the noninsertional tendon or an insertional bony prominence. The latter is often irritated by tight shoe counters.

Examination

Physical examination begins with gait analysis and observation of the patient in a standing position. Both feet should be unshod with the legs exposed to the level of the knee. This allows for the assessment of lower extremity alignment, as well as the presence of global and regional swelling. Gait analysis includes normal walking and also having patients walk on their forefeet and then on their heels. The former is particularly helpful in assessing the strength at the gastrocsoleus complex. Finally, it is particularly helpful to observe patients walking not only toward and away from the examiner (Figure 8-1), but also from the side as they walk past the examiner (Figure 8-2). The latter highlights dynamic collapse of the longitudinal arch and also early toe-off.

Next, the patient is examined while sitting or lying down (Table 8-2). This includes a thorough neurovascular examination including palpation of both the dorsalis pedis and posterior tibial pulses. Active and passive ankle and subtalar range of motion are also assessed. Normal ankle motion is approximately 20 degrees of dorsiflexion and 40 degrees of plantar flexion. It is essential to test ankle motion with the knee both flexed and extended. A positive Silfverskiold test is present when there is decreased ankle dorsiflexion only with the knee extended, and signifies a gastrocnemius contracture (Figure 8-3). If there is decreased dorsiflexion with the knee both flexed and extended, then an Achilles contracture is present. Muscle strength should be evaluated in both legs and is evaluated on a scale of 1 to 5. Next, the posterior heel, ankle, and hindfoot are

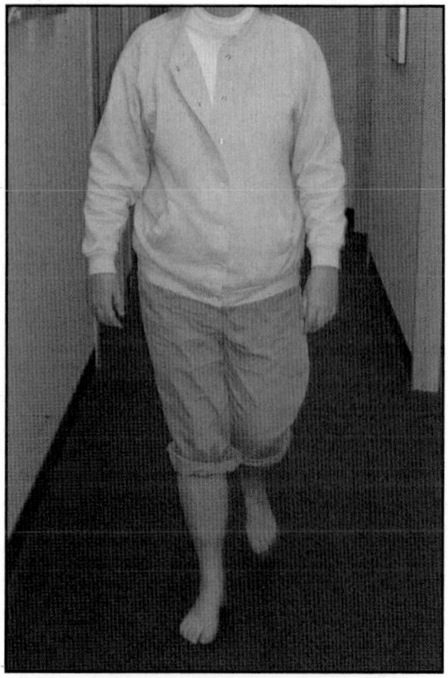

Figure 8-1. Gait analysis with the patient walking toward the examiner.

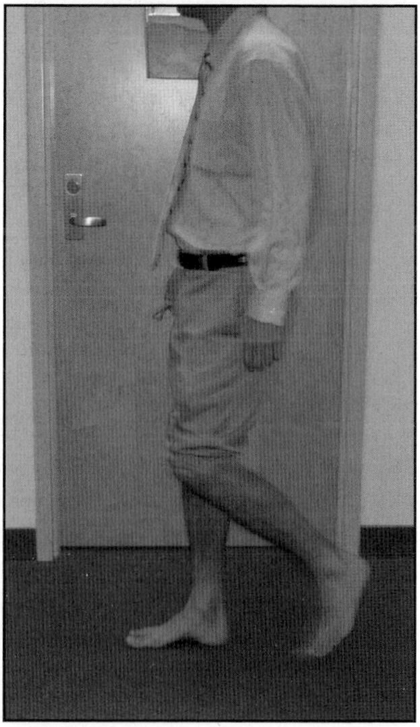

Figure 8-2. Gait analysis from the side with the patient walking past the examiner.

Table 8-2

Methods for Examination

Examination	*Technique*	*Illustration*	*Significance*
Ankle range of motion	Assess both active and passive motion	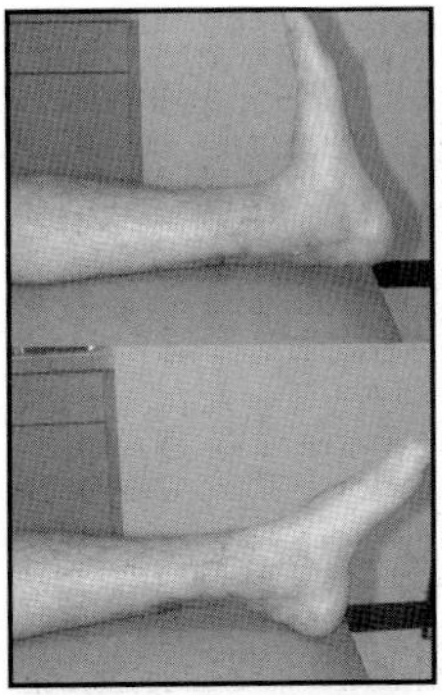	Normal is 20 degrees of dorsiflexion and 40 degrees of plantar flexion
Palpation	Focused examination of individual anatomic structures	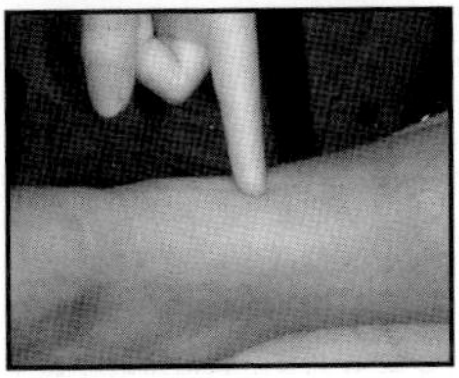	Specific diagnoses can usually be differentiated. Tendinosis is often nodular. Acute rupture demonstrates a gap in the tendon.
Thompson test	Observe passive ankle plantar flexion with manual calf compression	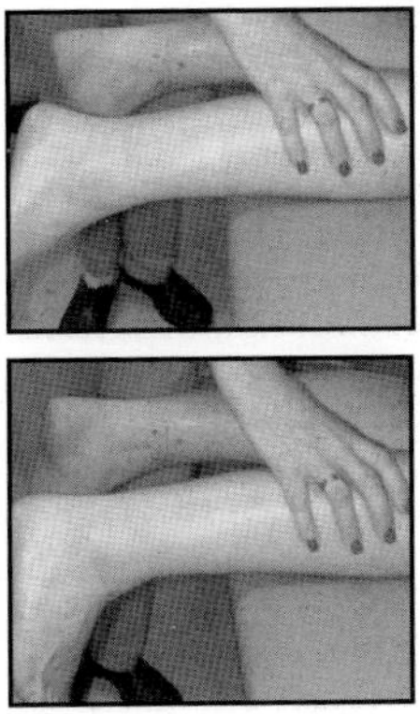	Positive (no ankle plantar flexion) with Achilles rupture, indicating discontinuity between the calf musculature and calcaneus.

(continued)

Table 8-2 (continued)

Methods for Examination

Examination	*Technique*	*Illustration*	*Significance*
Silfverskiold test	Assess ankle dorsiflexion with knee both flexed and extended	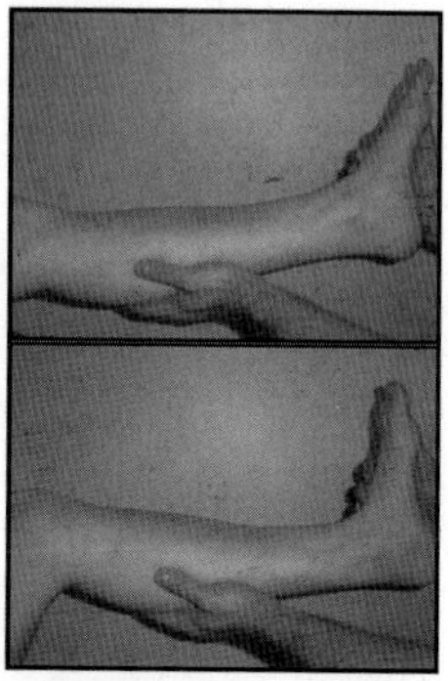	Positive if increased ankle dorsiflexion with knee flexed compared to extended, indicating presence of a gastrocnemius contracture
Calcaneal squeeze test	Manual compression of posterior calcaneal tuberosity	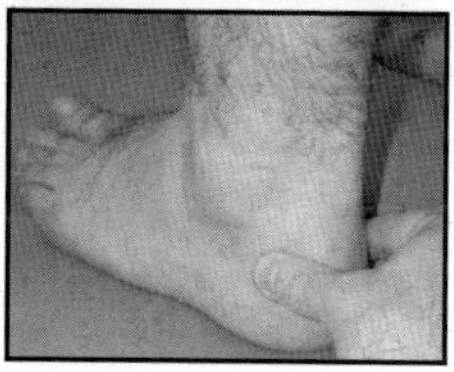	Tenderness is suggestive of calcaneal stress fracture

carefully palpated (Figure 8-4). Tenderness is often localized sufficiently so that a diagnosis can be confidently established. Palpation should include the insertional and noninsertional Achilles tendon, the retrocalcaneal bursa, the posterior calcaneal tuberosity, and the anatomic structures of both the posterolateral and posteromedial ankle. When palpating the Achilles tendon itself, tendon nodularity, thickening, and swelling should be noted.

In the setting of an acute Achilles tendon rupture, palpation usually reveals a gap in the tendon. In addition, a Thompson test should be performed.[6] With the patient either prone or kneeling on a chair, the posterior calf is manually compressed. The absence of passive ankle plantar flexion with this is consistent with discontinuity of the Achilles tendon (Figure 8-5).

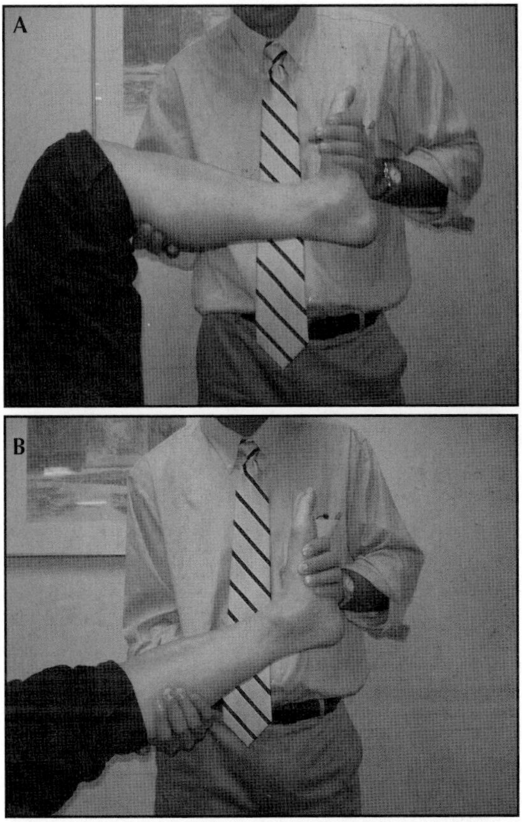

Figure 8-3. Positive Silfverskiold test. The ankle dorsiflexes past neutral with the knee flexed (A), but not with the knee extended (B).

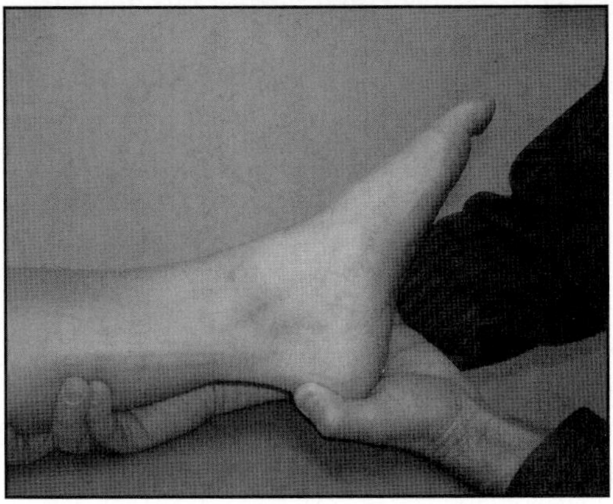

Figure 8-4. Palpation of the posterior heel region.

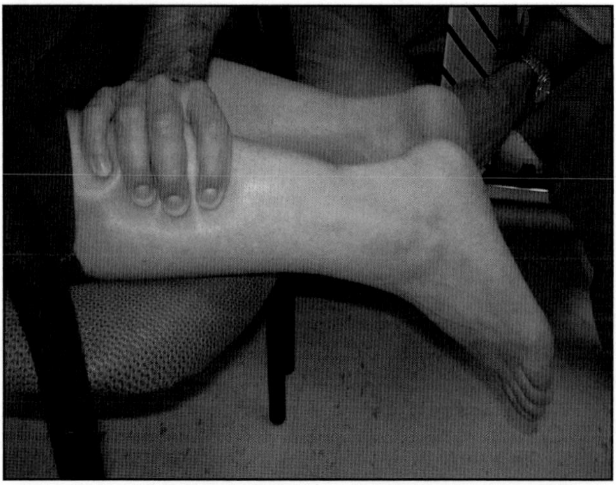

Figure 8-5. Normal Thompson test: Calf compression with an intact Achilles results in ankle plantar flexion.

Pathoanatomy

The Achilles tendon is a conjoined structure that inserts onto the posterior aspect of the calcaneus. It is formed proximally by the gastrocnemius and soleus muscles. Distal to the musculotendinous junction, the Achilles tendon has no true synovial sheath and is instead encased by a paratenon of varying thickness.[7,8] The blood supply of the tendon arises distally from calcaneal arterioles, proximally from intramuscular branches, and peripherally through the paratenon. A region of relative hypovascularity 2 to 6 cm proximal to the insertion has been described.[8] It is thought that this may predispose the tendon to degenerative change.

There are 2 bursa associated with the Achilles tendon. The retrocalcaneal bursa is a true bursa located between the posterior aspect of the calcaneal tuberosity and the anterior portion of the Achilles tendon. A second, more superficial bursa sometimes forms between the posterior aspect of the tendon and the subcutaneous tissues.[8]

The term *tendinosis* describes degeneration of a tendon. Macroscopically, the tendon shows thickening and areas of focal degeneration or partial tendon ruptures.

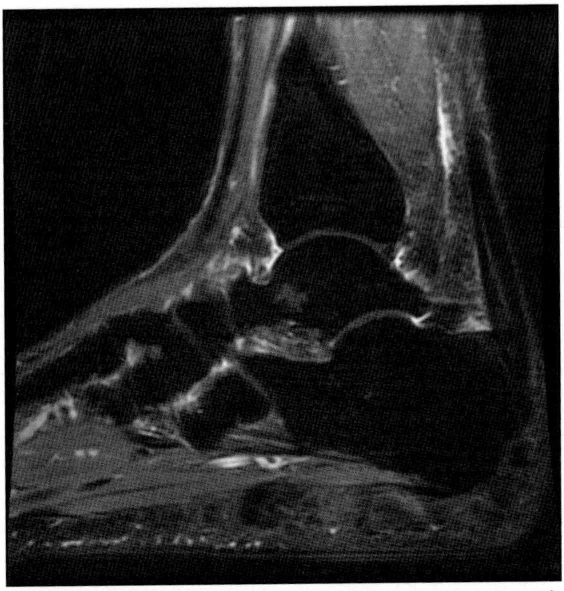

Figure 8-6. MRI demonstrating Achilles tendinosis with increased signal within the tendon.

Imaging

Patients with posterior heel pain typically undergo radiographic assessment with radiographs of the involved ankle. Three weight-bearing views—anteroposterior, mortise, and lateral—should be obtained. Thickening of the tendon is often visible. In addition, insertional and noninsertional calcifications can be detected. Finally, the ankle and hindfoot can be evaluated for such other pathology as fracture, arthritis, neoplasm, and the presence of an os trigonum.

With regard to advanced imaging, magnetic resonance imaging (MRI) is the most sensitive and accurate modality to confirm the diagnosis of tendinosis. A normal Achilles tendon is seen as low intensity signal on all MRI sequences, and a diseased tendon is typically seen as any increase in intratendinous signal intensity (Figure 8-6).[9] Ultrasound has recently gained popularity in the evaluation of Achilles tendon pathology.[10] It obviates the use of ionizing radiation and can be performed in the office setting. However, this modality is operator dependent with a substantial learning curve and does not image peritendinous structures as well as MRI.

Treatment

The initial treatment of both Achilles tendinitis and tendinosis should be nonoperative. There are numerous options including nonsteroidal anti-inflammatory medications, physical therapy, orthotics, heel lifts, night splints, extracorporeal shockwave, immobilization, and bracing. Physical therapy typically entails stretching, eccentric muscle exercises, and local modalities such as ultrasound and deep friction massage. The use of a night splint is particularly helpful to patients with morning pain. Temporary immobilization may be accomplished using a walking cast or pneumatic compression boot, while long-term bracing calls for either an ankle-foot orthosis or a custom leather gauntlet brace (eg, Arizona brace).

Of note, we do not recommend the use of steroid injections around the Achilles tendon because this may predispose the patient to subsequent tendon rupture.[11]

If symptoms persist beyond 3 to 6 months, surgery should be considered. Numerous procedures have been described. These typically include some combination of posterior calcaneal ostectomy, bursectomy, and tendon débridement (including intratendinous degeneration and calcifications). For refractory peritendinitis without tendinosis, normal saline or local anesthetic may be instilled between the tendon and the paratenon ("brisement"). Alternatively, paratenon excision has been reported to be successful in 70% to 100% of cases.[12] Cases in which there is advanced tendon degeneration may need augmentation utilizing a transfer of the flexor hallucis longus (FHL) tendon. Finally, cases with advanced tendinosis may require such radical débridement that a gap is created. This can be addressed by a fascial turn-down, V-Y musculotendinous advancement, or FHL transfer.

The treatment of an acute Achilles tendon rupture may be either operative or nonoperative. In general, the operative treatment of an acute rupture is indicated in young, active patients, in whom return to athletics is important. Although surgery minimizes the risk of re-rupture compared with nonoperative treatment (3.5% versus 12.6%), it has been associated with a higher risk of other complications, in particular wound problems.[13] These can be minimized with minimally invasive repairs and modern operative technique.[14]

The nonoperative treatment of acute Achilles rupture using cast immobilization has historically been reserved for elderly and sedentary individuals. The foot is initially immobilized in equinus for several weeks and then in neutral for several more weeks. While avoiding wound problems, cast immobilization increases the risk of re-rupture. More recently, other authors have reported improved results utilizing functional bracing, allowing early weight bearing and motion in special braces or fracture boots with incorporated heel lifts.[15,16]

Conclusion

Posterior heel pain is a common orthopedic complaint and, in the vast majority of cases, is associated with disorders of the Achilles tendon. The physical examination in these patients is usually straightforward, and appropriate treatment can be initiated without advanced imaging. Most patients will ultimately enjoy complete or near-complete relief with either operative or nonoperative management.

References

1. Habusta SF. Bilateral simultaneous rupture of the Achilles tendon. A rare traumatic injury. *Clin Orthop Relat Res*. 1995;(320):231-234.
2. Metzl J, Ahmad C, Levine W. The ruptured Achilles tendon: operative and non-operative treatment options. *Current Rev Musculoskelet Med*. 2008;1(2):161-164.
3. Puddu G, Ippolito E, Postacchini F. A classification of Achilles tendon disease. *Am J Sports Med*. 1976;4(4):145-150.
4. Ballas MT, Tytko J, Mannarino F. Commonly missed orthopedic problems. *Am Fam Physician*. 1998;57(2):267-274.
5. Akermark C. Difficulty in diagnosing total rupture of the Achilles tendon. *Lakartidningen*. 1992;89(44):3681-3683.
6. Thompson TC, Doherty JH. Spontaneous rupture of tendon of Achilles: a new clinical diagnostic test. *J Trauma*. 1962;2:126-129.
7. Dalton G. Achilles tendon rupture. *Foot Ankle*. 1996;1:225-236.
8. Coughlin M, Mann R, Saltzman C. *Surgery of the Foot and Ankle*. 8th ed. Philadephia, PA: Elsevier; 2007:1221-1261.

9. Deutsch AL, Mink JH. Magnetic resonance imaging of musculoskeletal injuries. *Radiol Clin North Am.* 1989;27(5):983-1002.
10. Reach JS, Nunley J. Ultrasound examination of the Achilles tendon. In: Nunly JA. *The Achilles Tendon: Treatment and Rehabilitation.* 2009;(2):17-23.
11. Metcalfe D, Achten J, Costa ML. Glucocorticoid injection in lesions of the Achilles tendon. *Foot Ankle Int.* 2009;30(7):661-665.
12. Coughlin M, Schon L, Mann R, Saltzman C. Disorders of Tendons. *Surgery of the Foot and Ankle.* 8th ed. Philadephia, PA: Elsevier; 2007:1149-1277.
13. Khan RJ, Fick D, Keogh A, Crawford J, Brammar T, Parker M. Treatment of acute Achilles tendon ruptures. A meta-analysis of randomized, controlled trials. *J Bone Joint Surg Am.* 2005;87(10):2202-2210.
14. Chiodo CP, Den Hartog B. Surgical strategies: acute Achilles rupture–open repair. *Foot Ankle Int.* 2008;29(1):114-118.
15. Feinblatt J, Graves S. Disorders of the anterior tibial, peroneal and Achilles tendons. In: Pinzur MS. *Orthopaedic Knowledge Update.* 4th ed. Rosemont: IL; American Academy of Orthopaedic Surgeons. 2008;115-133.
16. Costa ML, MacMillian K, Halliday D, et al. Randomised controlled trials of immediate weight-bearing mobilization for rupture of the tendo Achilles. *J Bone Joint Surg Br.* 2006; 88(1):69-77.

9

Fractures

Samir Mehta, MD

Introduction

The awareness and treatment of traumatic injuries of the foot and ankle have increased substantially over the past decade. With the increased effectiveness of first responders, greater motor vehicle safety features (eg, seat belts, airbags), and increased access to trauma centers, individuals are surviving their initial traumatic injury but are sustaining frequent and higher-energy foot and ankle injuries (Figure 9-1). One series revealed the poor outcome of polytrauma patients who sustained injuries to the foot and ankle, which led to a disproportionately lower clinical outcome score compared to similar patients without injuries to the distal limb.[1]

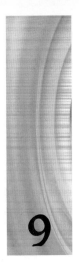

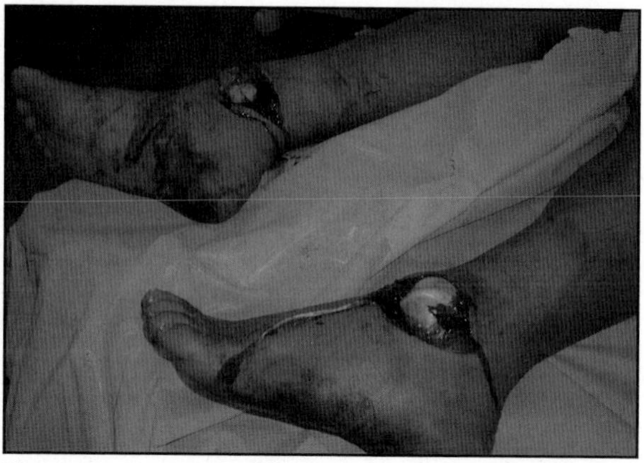

Figure 9-1. A 32-year-old female involved in a high-energy motor vehicle collision with isolated bilateral lower extremity open talus fracture-dislocations.

In addition to the increasing numbers of high-energy foot and ankle injuries, the aging population is contributing to the pool as well. Ankle fractures are the most common weight-bearing skeletal injury with the highest incidence in elderly women, many of whom are osteoporotic.[2] Fractures around the ankle typically involve only the lateral malleolus about 68% of the time, followed by bimalleolar injuries (25%), and trimalleolar fractures (7%). Despite limited soft tissue coverage, only 2% of ankle fractures are open. Unlike certain other fractures, there is little debate about the superiority of operative treatment over nonoperative management in the care of the majority of ankle fractures. On the other hand, despite their relative frequency, little is known about the epidemiology and outcomes of foot fractures. With advances in computed tomography (CT) and magnetic resonance imaging (MRI), the severity of foot fractures has been highlighted with particular attention being paid to the soft tissue anatomy along with osseous injury.

While less common than ankle and forefoot fractures, fractures of the hindfoot and midfoot are essential to identify and treat because missed injuries can lead to considerable long-term disability. Fracture of the calcaneus, talus, and Lisfranc's region can be difficult to treat given the complications associated with surgical management; however, nonoperative treatment of these injuries may also lead to suboptimal outcomes.

History

Most patients present with isolated foot and ankle fractures after low-energy injuries. Patients who sustain foot and ankle fractures as a result of high-energy trauma must be examined using Advanced Trauma Life Support principles because they may have other injuries as well. Injuries to the calcaneus and talus are often high energy and require a thorough assessment.

Understanding the mechanism of injury from the patient will often allow one to not only determine the energy of the injury, but also direct radiographic and physical examination. Axial loads to the limb, such as in a fall or during a motor vehicle collision, may be indicative of a calcaneus or talus fracture. A torsional or rotational mechanism of injury will likely result in an ankle fracture or Lisfranc's injury.

Due to the limited soft tissue envelope, patients will often describe swelling and pain directly over the region of injury and can often localize their pain due to the osseous disruption. In addition, patients should be asked about previous ankle or foot injuries, work status and occupation, and ability to cope with being non–weight-bearing for a period of time as most injuries—regardless of treatment—require some period of immobilization. In addition, it is important to take into account medical comorbidities such as vascular disease, diabetes, osteoporosis, smoking, steroid use, and previous surgeries as all of these may impact treatment.

Examination

Physical examination of an injured foot and ankle begins first with inspection of the soft tissue, palpation of the medial and lateral malleoli, and assessment of ligamentous stability. There may be an obvious deformity of the foot and/or ankle depending on the mechanism and energy of the injury. Patients typically have considerable discomfort with manipulation of the lower extremity and analgesia may be necessary to obtain an adequate examination. In the deformed lower extremity, immediate assessment of neurologic, vascular, and soft tissue structures should be made to determine if an emergent reduction is necessary. Compromised skin, diminished or absent pulses, or abnormal or lack of sensation in the dislocated or nonreduced limb should warrant an immediate reduction. Documentation of neurovascular status pre- and postreduction is essential.

The physical examination should include an extensive examination of the soft tissue coverage over the ankle and foot. Given the relative paucity of muscle around the distal extremity, fractures in this region may be open, and due diligence in examining for punctate (Type I) wounds is critical. Open injuries are rare but, if present, are usually medial in location and associated with lateral dislocation. The wounds are typically long (8 cm), linear, and tension-type failures often occurring in frail, thin, elderly skin.[3] They can usually be primarily closed. Furthermore, the limited soft tissue envelope is at risk for pressure necrosis by displaced fractures or dislocated joints, with rates as high as 12% being reported in the literature.[2]

A number of neurovascular structures and tendons run on both sides of the hindfoot, including the peroneal tendons and the sural nerve laterally and the posterior tibialis tendon, flexor digitorum longus tendon, and flexor hallucis longus tendons medially under the sustentaculum tali. Medially, the posterior tibial artery and the posterior tibial nerve are also at risk. An assessment of the dorsalis pedis and the posterior tibial artery should be performed by direct palpation and compared to the uninjured side. Differences in pulses warrant further examination such as an Ankle-Brachial Index with values less than 0.9 concerning for vascular injury.[4] Neurologic examination includes sensation over the dorsal and plantar surfaces of the foot as well as assessment of the motor function.

Certain examination maneuvers can be performed to assess specific injury patterns. Pain during palpation over the entire course of the fibula or pain with side-to-side compression of the tibia and fibula at least 5 cm over the joint may be indicative of a syndesmotic injury.[5] Other associated injuries can include fifth metatarsal or calcaneus fractures. The syndesmosis can be further evaluated through a stress examination of the ankle.[6] Particular interest should be paid to the spine in patients with an axial loading mechanism of injury that have either a calcaneus or talus fracture because there is a high associated rate of lumbar spine fractures in patients with this injury mechanism. In addition, high-energy or crush injuries of the foot should be monitored for compartment syndrome, with an incidence as high as 10% in calcaneus fractures. Patients with a suspected Lisfranc's fracture/dislocation often have tenderness with passive abduction and pronation of the forefoot with the hindfoot held fixed in the examiner's opposite hand or ecchymosis on the plantar surface of the foot.[7]

Pathoanatomy

The ankle joint is formed from the distal fibula, distal tibia, and talus. As the ankle dorsiflexes, the fibula rotates externally to accommodate the wider anterior talus. The tibia and fibula are connected by the inferior transverse ligament, which lies posteriorly below the inferior tibiofibular syndesmosis. The syndesmosis consists of the anterior and posterior tibiofibular ligaments and the interosseous ligament.[8] The tibiofibular complex is attached to the hindfoot medially by the deltoid and laterally by the calcaneofibular and posterior talofibular ligaments, which are quite strong and assist in fracture propagation. The Lauge-Hansen classification system is based on the position of the foot and the deforming force at the time of fracture.[9-12] By understanding the position of the foot, the forces applied across the region, and the ligamentous stabilizers, predictable fracture patterns develop—supination-external rotation (SER), pronation-external-rotation, pronation-abduction, and supination-adduction. SER injuries are the most common, resulting in an oblique fracture of the fibula. As the energy of the injury goes "around" the ankle, the SER pattern can include a medial malleolus fracture (transverse) and a posterior malleolus component as well. Syndesmotic injuries are most common in displaced Weber B fractures. The Weber classification refers to the location of the fracture line in the fibula relative to the syndesmosis. Weber A fractures are below, Weber B fractures are at, and Weber C fractures are above the syndesmosis.

Fractures of the talar neck are often due to axial load with foot dorsiflexed. Two-thirds of the talus is covered with articular cartilage, there are no tendons or muscles that originate

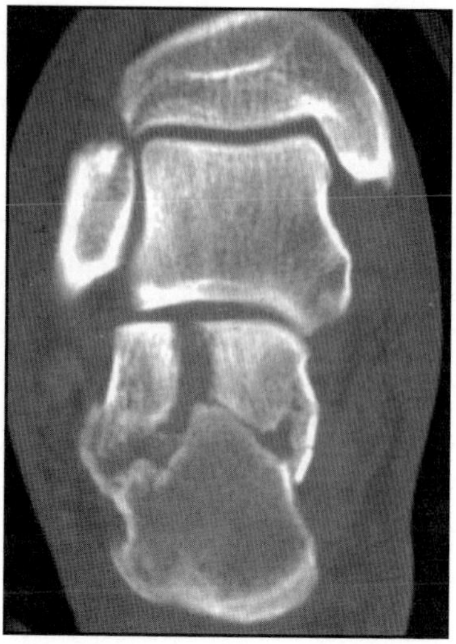

Figure 9-2. CT scan of the calcaneus showing the primary fracture line through the posterior facet as well as the lateral wall blowout.

from or insert into it, and the blood supply is relatively poor, so avascular necrosis is a significant problem after fracture. The superior aspect of the talus articulates with the tibial plafond and the medial and lateral malleoli, while the inferior aspect has 3 facets articulating with the calcaneus. The blood supply comes from 3 arteries—posterior tibial artery branch to the tarsal canal, artery of the tarsal sinus, and arteries perforating through the deltoid—which are at extreme risk with displaced fractures of the talar neck.

The anatomy of the calcaneus is complex and fractures can occur in all parts of the bone. The anterior, posterior, and middle facets articulate with the talus which can act as a wedge driving into the calcaneus with a high-energy axial load. Intra-articular fractures of the calcaneus often involve the posterior facet and may also result in injury to other facets, the calcaneal tuberosity, and the calcaneocuboid joint.[13] The primary fracture line, which runs from anterolateral to posteromedial, is made by the lateral process of the talus being driven downward. The distance of this line from the sustentaculum tali ("constant fragment") can vary. As the talus is driven further into the calcaneus, the posterolateral fragment can become comminuted and the lateral wall of the calcaneus is "blown out" (Figure 9-2). The calcaneus is often flattened, short, and

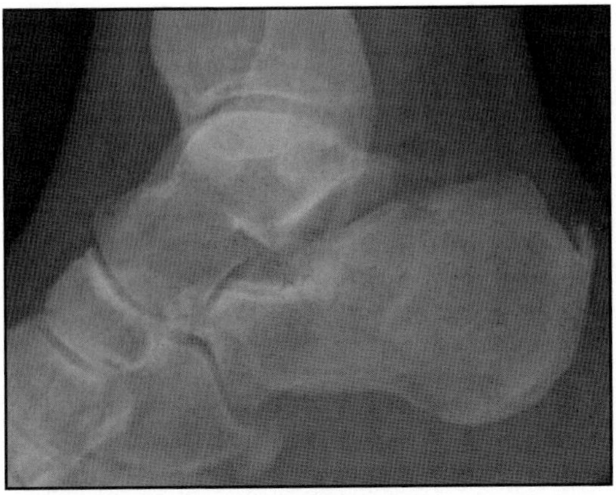

Figure 9-3. Lateral radiograph of a calcaneus fracture revealing a flat Böhler angle and shortening of the calcaneus.

in varus (Figure 9-3).[13] Extra-articular calcaneus fractures are also important, particularly those of the posterior tuberosity where the soft tissue posteriorly can be compromised by the pull of the Achilles (Figure 9-4).[14]

Dislocation of the tarsometatarsal (Lisfranc's) joint usually occurs due to an axial load to the dorsiflexed midfoot or in a twisting injury to the midfoot. The stability of the joint is gained from the strong intraosseous ligaments and the fact that the second metatarsal articulates with the medial cuneiform proximal to the articulation of the medial and lateral cuneiforms of the first and third metatarsals. Three basic dislocation patterns (homolateral, isolated, and divergent) have been described based on the direction of the dislocation and the extent of ligamentous injury (Figure 9-5). Up to 80% of Lisfranc's injuries are associated with other fractures in the foot.

Imaging

Radiographs of the ankle include anteroposterior (AP), lateral, and mortise views. Radiographs alone are often all that is needed to diagnose ankle fractures (Table 9-1). The lateral view allows assessment of posterior malleolar fractures, AP subluxation of the talus under the tibia, distal fibula translation, or a talus fracture. If there is concern about articular

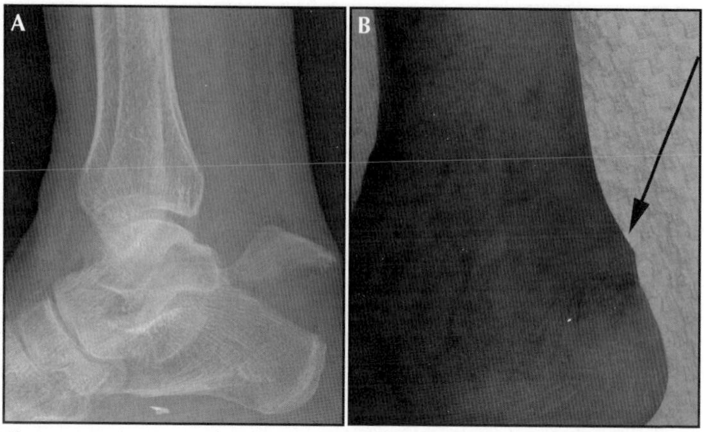

Figure 9-4. (A) Lateral radiograph of the calcaneus showing a posterior tuberosity avulsion with significant displacement due to the pull of the Achilles tendon. (B) Clinical picture showing skin tenting from avulsed tuberosity piece (black arrow) necessitating urgent reduction.

Figure 9-5. AP radiograph of the foot with homolateral Lisfranc's fracture dislocation after direct trauma to the foot during a rock concert.

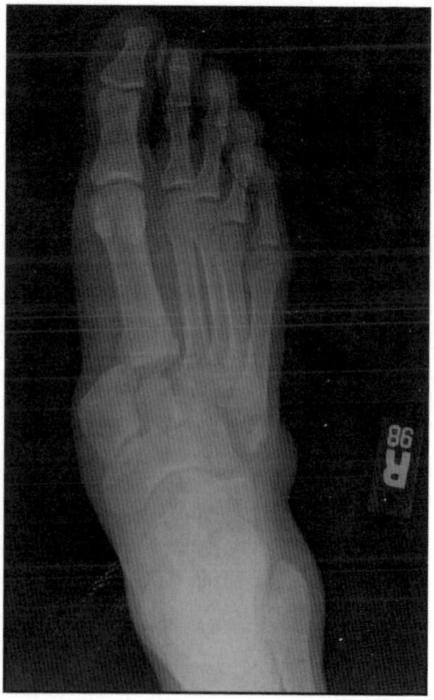

Table 9-1

Helpful Hints for Addressing Syndesmosis

Issue	*Options*
Preoperative assessment	Gravity stress
	Stress external rotation
Intraoperative assessment	Lateral fibular stress (Cotton test)
	Stress external rotation
	Comparison to uninjured side on lateral view
Reduction	Percutaneous clamp application
	Manual (using hands)
	Direct visualization (anterior exposure)
Fixation	3.5-mm fully-threaded screw (1 or 2)
	4.5-mm fully-threaded screw (1 or 2)
	Dynamic stabilization (eg, "Tightrope," FiberWire)
	Bioabsorbable screw fixation
Number of cortices	Three
	Four
	Static screw (not lag technique)
Postoperative regimen	No weight bearing for at least 8 to 10 weeks
	Discuss screw removal with patient (not essential)
	Breakage
	Loosening
	Backing out

comminution, complex fracture patterns, or an irreducible ankle fracture/dislocation, a CT scan may provide additional information. The use of MRI provides little information in terms of osseus abnormalities but may assess the syndesmosis.

Diagnosing a concomitant syndesmotic injury is essential (Table 9-2).[15] The AP radiograph will visualize tibiofibular

Table 9-2

Methods for Obtaining Appropriate Radiographs of the Foot and Ankle

View	*Position of the Limb*	*Location of the Beam*	*Notes*
Mortise view	Internal rotation 15 degrees	Directly AP over the ankle	Important to obtain a symmetric joint space
Gravity stress view	Affected limb lateral on stretcher	Positioned for an AP of the ankle (with ankle to the side)	Patient placed in lateral decubitus with the affected side down
Stress external rotation view	Internal rotation 15 degrees	Directly AP over the ankle	Ten to 15 pounds of external rotation force applied to forefoot while holding tibia
Canale view	Plantarflex ankle and 15 degrees of pronation	AP of the foot with the beam entering at 15 degrees from the vertical plane	May require adduction of the midfoot as well
Broden's view	Foot internal rotation 20 degrees; varying degrees of plantar flexion from 10 to 40	Anterior to posteriorly directed beam	Assesses posterior facet
Axial (Harris) heel view	Second toe in line with tibia; foot fully dorsiflexed	Image intensifier should be in lateral position and beam should be at 45 degrees to calcaneus	Will provide assessment of hindfoot varus or valgus

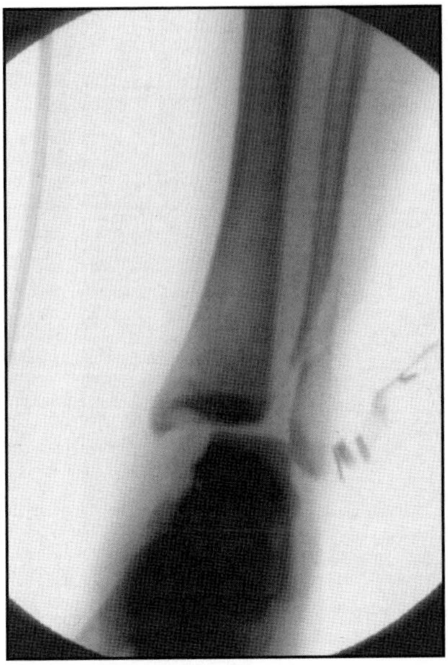

Figure 9-6. Intraoperative image intensifier view of an ankle fracture in a football player revealing no tibiofibular overlap, increased clear space, talar tilt, and medial joint space widening.

overlap (greater than 10 mm is normal, with less overlap indicative of syndesmotic injury), tibiofibular clear space (less than 5 mm is normal, with more indicative of a syndesmotic injury), and talar tilt (less than 2 mm is normal) (Figure 9-6). Any medial joint space widening on the mortise view is abnormal, as is a talocrural ankle of less than 8 degrees or greater than 15 degrees. If there is less than 1 mm of tibiofibular overlap on the mortise view, one should consider syndesmotic injury. Stress views (external rotation or gravity) can evaluate the integrity of the syndesmosis. Ultimately, if operative fixation of ankle factures is undertaken, intraoperative assessment with lateral fibular stress (Cotton test) or stress external rotation should be performed.

Imaging of the talus includes a foot and ankle series as well as a Canale view (ankle in plantar flexion with 15 degrees of pronation and the beam entering at 15 degrees from the vertical plane). A CT scan (Figure 9-7) can be useful to further delineate injury pattern and MRI can be performed primarily to assess for complications such as avascular necrosis (AVN). The Hawkins classification system, which is predictive of AVN, is used to describe these injuries. Type I fractures are

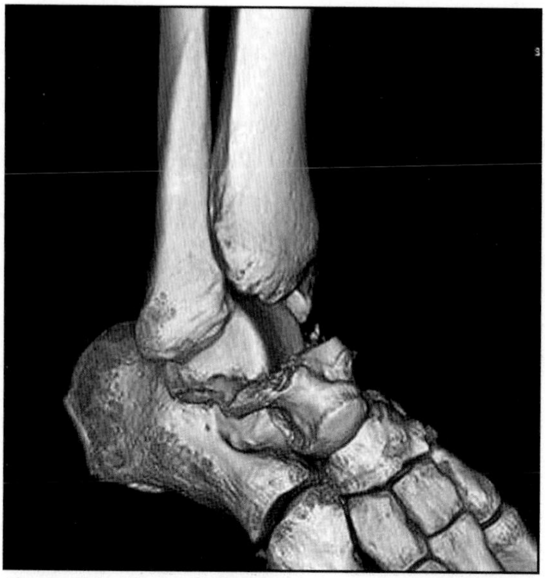

Figure 9-7. Three-dimensional CT reconstruction view in a displaced talar neck fracture after a fall from a motorcycle.

nondisplaced. Type II fractures are associated with subluxation or dislocation of the subtalar joint. Type III fractures include dislocation of the subtalar joint with associated dislocation or subluxation of the ankle joint. Type IV fractures include those where the talar head is dislocated from the navicular.

Plain radiographs will identify most calcaneus fractures. Lateral radiographs can reveal changes in Böhler angle (normally 20 to 40 degrees) and the critical angle of Gissane. A flat Böhler angle indicates posterior facet involvement. A Broden's view examines the posterior facet and is taken with the foot position in 20 degrees of internal rotation with 10 to 40 degrees of plantar flexion. Axial radiographs assess varus/valgus angulation of the calcaneus with the image taken as a 45-degree axial of the heel with the second toe in line with the tibia (normal alignment is 10 degrees of valgus). The CT scan, however, is a better tool for assessment of the posterior facet and extent of comminution and should be performed perpendicular to the posterior facet with sagittal cuts parallel to the plantar aspect of foot. The Sanders classification for calcaneus

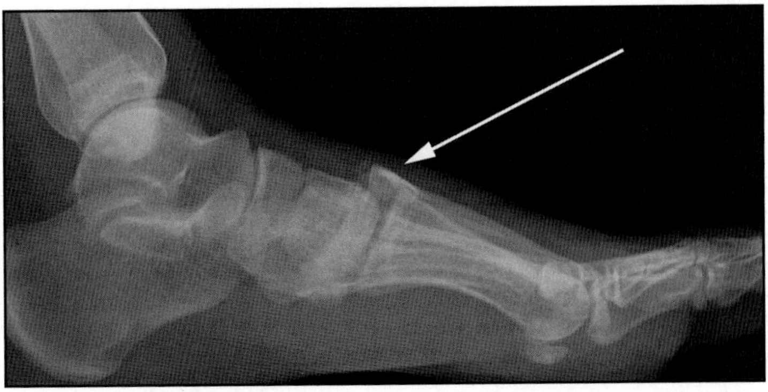

Figure 9-8. Lateral radiograph of the foot showing a step-off (white arrow) along the dorsal surface, suggesting a possible Lisfranc's injury.

fractures is based on the number of location of fractures lines on the CT scan.[16]

Suspected Lisfranc's injuries can be assessed with plain radiographs. An AP radiograph of the foot should show alignment of the medial margin of the second metatarsal base and medial margin of the medial cuneiform. An oblique radiograph should show alignment of the medial base of the fourth metatarsal and medial margin of the cuboid. On the lateral x-ray, the dorsal surface of the first and second metatarsals should be level to the corresponding cuneiforms (Figure 9-8). Standing stress films may demonstrate diastasis. In patients without obvious plain film changes, a CT or MRI scan may reveal displacement at the base of the second metatarsal or rupture of the interosseous ligaments.[17]

Treatment

In general, fractures of the foot and ankle often have a related soft-tissue injury. The patient's soft tissue swelling should dictate timing of intervention if surgery is indicated. Early operative management through swollen soft tissue only further traumatizes the soft-tissue envelope and can lead to complications such as infection and wound dehiscence. While there are certain injuries requiring emergent treatment, such as irreducible dislocations, displaced posterior calcaneal

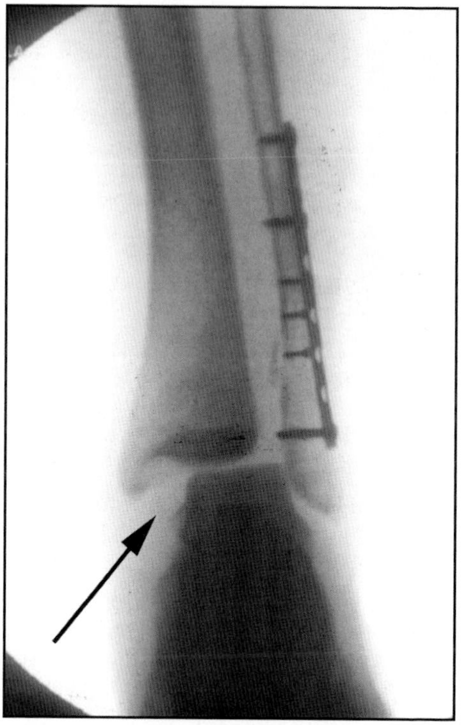

Figure 9-9. Fluoroscopic AP image of the ankle after fixation of the lateral malleolus with minifragment lag screws and a one-third tubular neutralization plate. Despite anatomic reduction of the fibula, stress external rotation reveals a widened syndesmosis and increased medial clear space (black arrow).

tuberosity fractures, and open fractures, most injuries of the foot and ankle can be treated in a delayed fashion once the soft tissue has acquiesced. Clinically, this is often measured by the presence of "wrinkles" in the soft tissue. If the soft tissue is severely compromised, external fixation may be applied to temporize until definite management can be performed. This may be necessary in high-energy injuries or open fractures.

Fractures of the ankle that are nondisplaced, minimally displaced, or stable can be managed nonoperatively with a brace or cast. Weight bearing is based on surgeon and patient comfort. Patients should be monitored closely to look for displacement, which may indicate the need for surgical stabilization. Displaced fractures of the ankle or fractures resulting in instability require anatomic reduction and fixation. The most common technique for fixation of the lateral malleolus involves interfragmentary lag screw fixation with a protection plate (Figure 9-9). Alternatively, a posterolateral plate can be applied to provide buttress fixation of the lateral malleolus.[18] Medial malleolar fractures are best fixed with open reduction and lag screw fixation across the fracture site. The posterior malleolus has gained significant attention. Smaller posterior malleolar fractures may reduce with fixation of the lateral malleolus. Displaced fractures, subluxation of the talus, or large fragments (20% to 33% of the articular surface) necessitate fixation of the posterior malleolus.[19,20] Fixation of the posterior malleolus can be performed percutaneously with anterior-posterior lag screws or posterior-anterior lag screws. However, for larger or comminuted fragments, an open reduction through a posterolateral exposure with buttress fixation may be warranted.[21]

Syndesmotic injury should be assessed after fixation of the osseous injury.[8] Fixation of the syndesmosis has been greatly debated. There is general agreement that the syndesmosis must be anatomically reduced and stabilized. Reduction of the syndesmosis can be performed closed with clamp reduction or open with direct visualization of the syndesmosis.[22] Once reduced, the syndesmosis can be secured with 1 or 2 fully-threaded large fragment or small fragment screws inserted from lateral to medial across 3 of 4 cortices approximately 1 in from the articular surface (Figure 9-10).

Nondisplaced fractures of the talus (Hawkins I) can be treated nonoperatively for 10 to 12 weeks with a non–weight-bearing cast. Displaced talar neck fractures require reduction and fixation. Timing of treatment has been debated. Reduction of dislocations must be performed emergently, which may limit the development of AVN. However, fixation may be performed in delayed fashion assuming accurate reduction.[23] Fixation can be performed with percutaneous techniques using anterior-to-posterior or posterior-to-anterior screw fixation. However, percutaneous treatment is associated with varus malreduction, which can be problematic long term. Open reduction and rigid fixation through anterolateral and anteromedial exposures allow for direct visualization of the talar neck. Fixation can be performed with screws alone or with mini-fragment plate application (see Figure 9-10).[24] Avascular necrosis rates vary from less than 10% in Hawkins type I to 90% to 100% in Hawkins type IV injuries. Treatment of avascular necrosis with arthrodesis is based on symptoms including degenerative changes of the subtalar or tibiotalar joints.

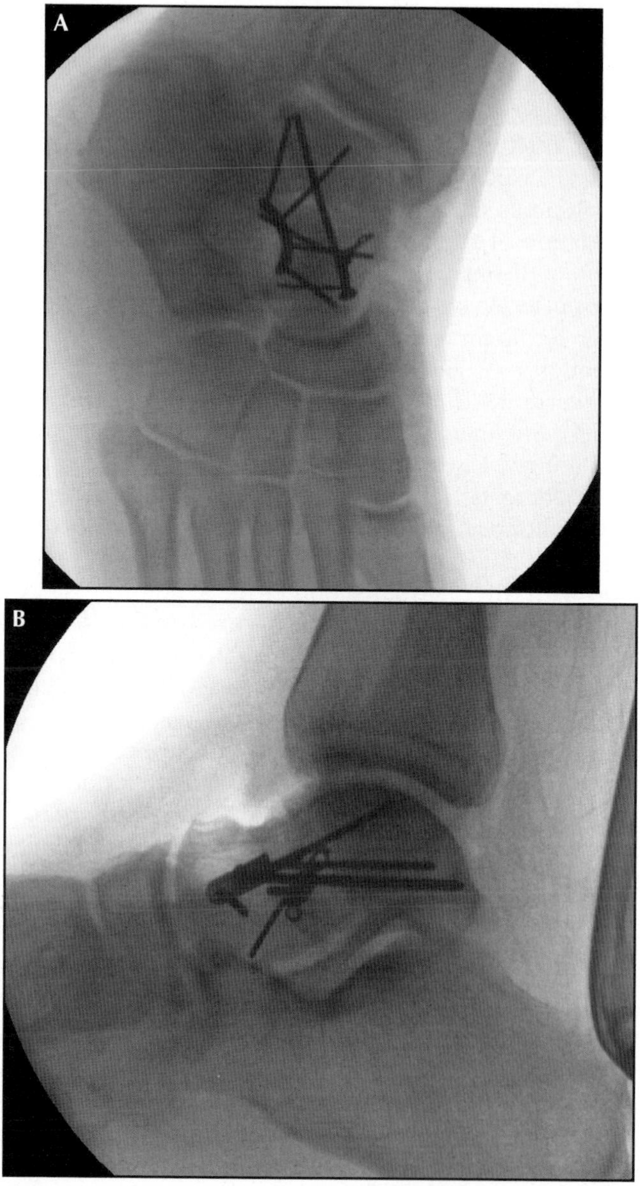

Figure 9-10. Intraoperative fluoroscopic (A) Canale view and (B) lateral view of the talus in the previous patient with reduction of the comminuted talar neck fracture via anteromedial and anterolateral exposures followed by fixation with mini-fragment plates and lag screws.

The treatment of intra-articular calcaneal fractures continues to be debated, but recent literature has supported fixation of displaced injuries. Nonoperative management often leads to chronic pain, limited weight bearing and mobility, and difficulty with post-traumatic reconstruction. Operative treatment includes open reduction and rigid internal fixation through an extensile lateral exposure with reduction of the articular surface, bone grafting, and stabilization via calcaneus-specific fixed angle (locking) plates (Figure 9-11).[13] Open exposure should be performed once soft tissue on the lateral side has wrinkles, which can take anywhere from 7 to 21 days. Complications of open treatment include wound infection due to the poor soft tissue envelope and the extensile nature of the exposure, leading to osteomyelitis. This is particularly concerning in patients who smoke, are vasculopaths, or have diabetes.[25,26] Increasing utilization of percutaneous reduction techniques has been promoted in this difficult patient population, limiting the soft tissue insult of the surgery, but also conceding the lack of direct articular reduction.[27] Percutaneous techniques should be employed within 48 to 72 hours after injury while the fragments are still mobile. Despite anatomic articular reduction, chondral injury in the subtalar joint can impact patient outcomes particularly with weight bearing on uneven ground and stair climbing. Most extra-articular calcaneus fractures can be treated nonoperatively. The exception to this is the posterior tuberosity fracture of the calcaneus where the soft tissue over the posterior aspect of the calcaneus can be compromised. In this case, urgent reduction of the fragment through either percutaneous or open techniques is warranted.[14] In patients who develop arthrosis or have severe pain or lack of mobility, subtalar arthrodesis may be performed.

Treatment of nondisplaced Lisfranc's injuries involves casting for 6 to 8 weeks. Displaced dislocations should be managed with open reduction and internal fixation with interfragmentary screws, plates, and/or Kirschner wires after an anatomic reduction (Figure 9-12). Some authors have suggested primary arthrodesis rather than fixation.[28,29] Missed Lisfranc's injuries or injuries without an associated fracture have poor prognosis, with late midfoot collapse a common sequela. Post-traumatic arthritis and planovalgus deformity are common and may

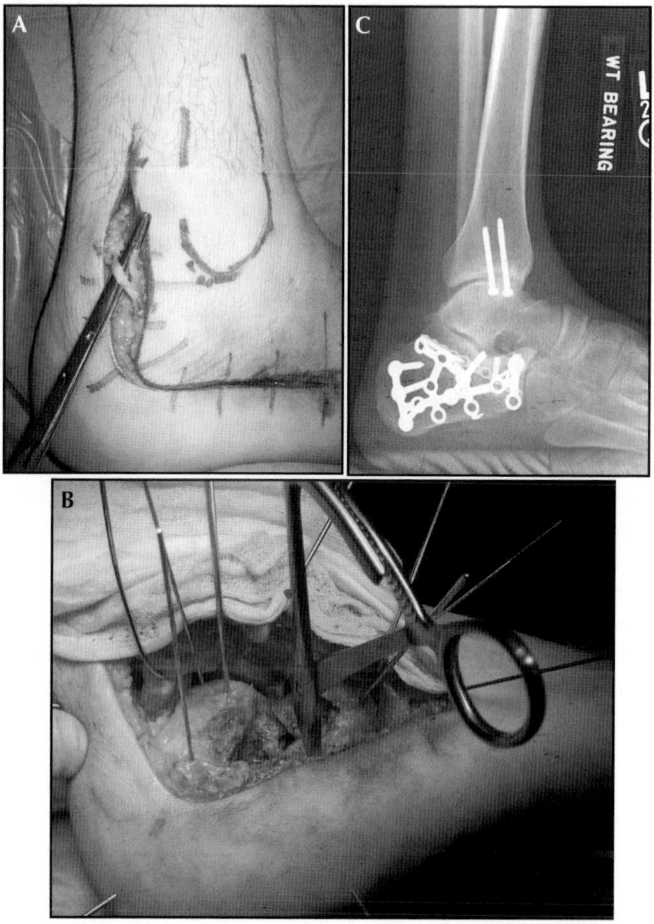

Figure 9-11. (A) Clinical picture of the surgical incision necessary for an extensile exposure to the calcaneus. The sural nerve has been identified in the proximal limb of the incision. (B) Via the extensile lateral exposure, the flap has been raised. It is kept out of the surgical field using Kirschner wires in a "no-touch" technique to maintain its viability. Visualization of the posterior facet, lateral wall, and calcaneocuboid joint, amongst other anatomy, is easily possible. In addition, application of reduction aids, provisional fixation, and implants is possible through this exposure. (C) Lateral radiograph of the calcaneus after fixation with a laterally based fixed angle implant showing restoration of Böhler angle, calcaneal length, and the posterior facet.

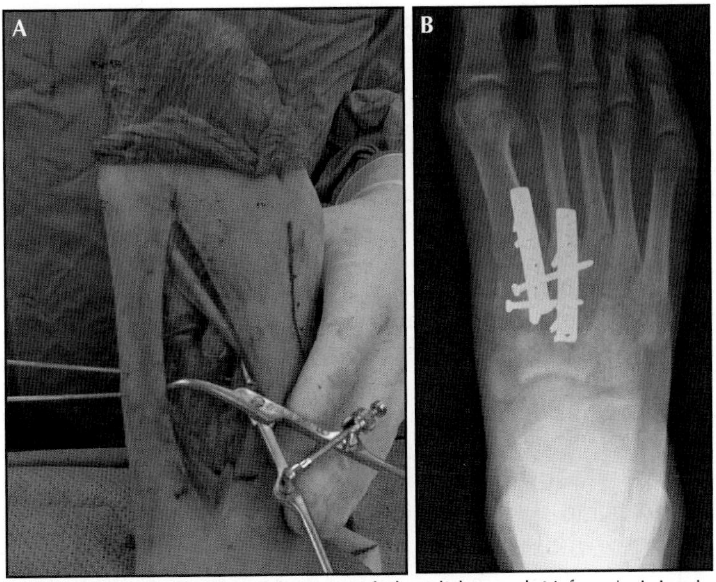

Figure 9-12. (A) Open reduction of the dislocated Lisfranc's joint in the previous patient. Via an open exposure, the severity of the injury can be better understood and an anatomic reduction can be obtained. (B) Postoperative AP radiograph showing fixation of the Lisfranc's with mini-fragment plates and screws in an effort to obtain and maintain an anatomic reduction.

occur in up to 50% of patients. Symptomatic post-traumatic arthritis may be treated with arthrodesis.

Postoperative management of operatively managed foot and ankle fractures often involves non–weight-bearing for at least 6 weeks and up to 12 weeks for calcaneus, talus, and Lisfranc's injuries. Range of motion can be started as early as 2 weeks once the soft tissue has healed. Protected weight bearing is begun with radiographic and clinical signs of healing. Recovery can continue up to 1 year after treatment with physiotherapy often necessary.[30]

Conclusion

Injuries of the foot and ankle are ever increasing in number. Accurate diagnosis is essential in developing a treatment plan. Certain injuries can be quite obvious, such as the dislocated ankle fracture. However, others are more subtle, such as the Lisfranc's injury, and often missed. These injuries can lead to significant disability long term. Most injuries of the foot and ankle, if they are reduced, can be managed in a delayed fashion. Compartment syndrome, open wounds, and soft-tissue or neurovascular compromise require immediate attention. Anatomic reduction has the potential to improve clinical outcomes, but the soft tissue component is critical as well. Early and aggressive range of motion may limit postoperative stiffness, but most patients have residual difficulty with high-demand activities particularly in higher-energy injury patterns.

References

1. Turchin DC, Schemitsch EH, McKee MD, Waddell JP. Do foot injuries significantly affect the functional outcome of multiply injured patients? *J Orthop Trauma*. 1999;13(1):1-4.
2. Hasselman CT, Vogt MT, Stone KL, Cauley JA, Conti SF. Foot and ankle fractures in elderly white women. Incidence and risk factors. *J Bone Joint Surg Am*. 2003;85-A(5):820-824.
3. Mehta S, Mirza AJ, Dunbar RP, Barei DP, Benirschke SK. A staged treatment plan for the management of Type II and Type IIIA open calcaneus fractures. *J Orthop Trauma*. 2010;24(3):142-147.
4. Mills WJ, Barei DP, McNair P. The value of the ankle-brachial index for diagnosing arterial injury after knee dislocation: a prospective study. *J Trauma*. 2004;56(6):1261-1265.
5. Alonso A, Khoury L, Adams R. Clinical tests for ankle syndesmosis injury: reliability and prediction of return to function. *J Orthop Sports Phys Ther*. 1998;27(4):276-284.
6. Schock HJ, Pinzur M, Manion L, Stover M. The use of gravity or manual-stress radiographs in the assessment of supination-external rotation fractures of the ankle. *J Bone Joint Surg Br*. 2007;89(8):1055-1059.
7. Ross G, Cronin R, Hauzenblas J, Juliano P. Plantar ecchymosis sign: a clinical aid to diagnosis of occult Lisfranc's tarsometatarsal injuries. *J Orthop Trauma*. 1996;10(2):119-122.
8. Wuest TK. Injuries to the Distal Lower Extremity Syndesmosis. *J Am Acad Orthop Surg*. 1997;5(3):172-181.

9. Lauge-Hansen N. Fractures of the ankle. II. Combined experimental-surgical and experimental-roentgenologic investigations. *Arch Surg.* 1950;60(5):957-985.
10. Lauge-Hansen N. Fractures of the ankle. IV. Clinical use of genetic roentgen diagnosis and genetic reduction. *AMA Arch Surg.* 1952;64(4):488-500.
11. Lauge-Hansen N. Fractures of the ankle. V. Pronation-dorsiflexion fracture. *AMA Arch Surg.* 1953;67(6):813-820.
12. Lauge-Hansen N. Fractures of the ankle. III. Genetic roentgenologic diagnosis of fractures of the ankle. *Am J Roentgenol Radium Ther Nucl Med.* 1954;71(3):456-471.
13. Barei DP, Bellabarba C, Sangeorzan BJ, Benirschke SK. Fractures of the calcaneus. *Orthop Clin North Am.* 2002;33(1):263-285, x.
14. Gardner MJ, Nork SE, Barei DP, Kramer PA, Sangeorzan BJ, Benirschke SK. Secondary soft tissue compromise in tongue-type calcaneus fractures. *J Orthop Trauma.* 2008;22(7):439-445.
15. Ostrum RF, De Meo P, Subramanian R. A critical analysis of the anterior-posterior radiographic anatomy of the ankle syndesmosis. *Foot Ankle Int.* 1995;16(3):128-131.
16. Sanders R, Fortin P, DiPasquale T, Walling A. Operative treatment in 120 displaced intraarticular calcaneal fractures. Results using a prognostic computed tomography scan classification. *Clin Orthop Relat Res.* 1993(290):87-95.
17. Raikin SM, Elias I, Dheer S, Besser MP, Morrison WB, Zoga AC. Prediction of midfoot instability in the subtle Lisfranc's injury. Comparison of magnetic resonance imaging with intraoperative findings. *J Bone Joint Surg Am.* 2009;91(4):892-899.
18. Wissing JC, van Laarhoven CJ, van der Werken C. The posterior antiglide plate for fixation of fractures of the lateral malleolus. *Injury.* 1992;23(2):94-96.
19. Gardner MJ, Brodsky A, Briggs SM, Nielson JH, Lorich DG. Fixation of posterior malleolar fractures provides greater syndesmotic stability. *Clin Orthop Relat Res.* 2006;447:165-171.
20. Tejwani NC, Pahk B, Egol KA. Effect of posterior malleolus fracture on outcome after unstable ankle fracture. *J Trauma.* 2010;69(3):666-669.
21. van den Bekerom MP, Haverkamp D, Kloen P. Biomechanical and clinical evaluation of posterior malleolar fractures. A systematic review of the literature. *J Trauma.* 2009;66(1):279-284.
22. Miller AN, Carroll EA, Parker RJ, Boraiah S, Helfet DL, Lorich DG. Direct visualization for syndesmotic stabilization of ankle fractures. *Foot Ankle Int.* 2009;30(5):419-426.
23. Vallier HA, Nork SE, Barei DP, Benirschke SK, Sangeorzan BJ. Talar neck fractures: results and outcomes. *J Bone Joint Surg Am.* 2004;86-A(8):1616-1624.
24. Charlson MD, Parks BG, Weber TG, Guyton GP. Comparison of plate and screw fixation and screw fixation alone in a comminuted talar neck fracture model. *Foot Ankle Int.* 2006;27(5):340-343.

25. Folk JW, Starr AJ, Early JS. Early wound complications of operative treatment of calcaneus fractures: analysis of 190 fractures. *J Orthop Trauma.* 1999;13(5):369-372.
26. Watson TS. Soft tissue complications following calcaneal fractures. *Foot Ankle Clin.* 2007;12(1):107-123.
27. DeWall M, Henderson CE, McKinley TO, Phelps T, Dolan L, Marsh JL. Percutaneous reduction and fixation of displaced intra-articular calcaneus fractures. *J Orthop Trauma.* 2010;24(8):466-472.
28. Henning JA, Jones CB, Sietsema DL, Bohay DR, Anderson JG. Open reduction internal fixation versus primary arthrodesis for lisfranc's injuries: a prospective randomized study. *Foot Ankle Int.* 2009;30(10):913-922.
29. Ly TV, Coetzee JC. Treatment of primarily ligamentous Lisfranc's joint injuries: primary arthrodesis compared with open reduction and internal fixation. A prospective, randomized study. *J Bone Joint Surg Am.* 2006;88(3):514-520.
30. Lin CW, Moseley AM, Refshauge KM. Rehabilitation for ankle fractures in adults. *Cochrane Database Syst Rev.* 2008(3):CD005595.

10

Foot and Ankle Arthritis

Eric Breitbart, MD; Wayne Berberian, MD; and Sheldon Lin, MD

Introduction

Arthritis is among the leading causes of disability in the United States. While most prevalent in the elderly, it can occur at any age, leading to severe morbidity and a lifetime of chronic pain. Foot and ankle arthritis, while approximately 9 times less common than hip or knee arthritis, affects millions of Americans.[1-4] Arthritis in the foot and ankle can be subdivided by location and etiology. In terms of location, the most common sites include the tibiotalar joint, the 3 joints of the hindfoot (subtalar, calcaneocuboid, and talonavicular), the metatarsocuneiform joint, and the first metatarsophalangeal (MTP) joint. The most common causes of foot and ankle

Hurwitz SR, Parekh SG. *Musculoskeletal Examination of the Foot and Ankle: Making the Complex Simple* (pp. 179-195). © 2012 SLACK Incorporated.

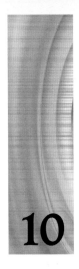

arthritis include post-traumatic arthritis (70% to 80%), inflammatory arthritis (10% to 15%), and primary osteoarthritis (7% to 15%), with infection and tumor comprising less than 1% of the etiology.[1-5] This epidemiology differs from the majority of joints, including the hip and knee, in which primary osteoarthritis, due to long-term overuse and stress in combination with the aging process, is the primary cause.[1-5]

Although not comprising the majority of cases of arthritis in the foot and ankle, pain in the foot and ankle is often the initial complaint of patients with rheumatoid arthritis (RA), with the prevalence of forefoot deformities in adults with chronic RA reported to approach 90%.[6-12] In RA, the prevalence of midfoot and hindfoot symptoms is about half that of forefoot and ankle symptoms, but significantly increases with duration of the disease.[7,8] Studies have demonstrated that over 75% of patients with RA have MTP joint subluxation in digits 2 to 5 (claw/hammer toe) and over 70% of patients have a hallux valgus deformity.[7,13] Because of the complexity and severity of deformities in RA, along with multijoint involvement, these patients may prove the most difficult for the orthopedic surgeon to treat.

History

Taking a strong history is fundamental in reaching a final diagnosis and treatment plan (Table 10-1). Since the most common cause of foot and ankle arthritis is post-traumatic in origin, a history of trauma to the joint should be ascertained, as well as any relevant past procedures (eg, open reduction internal fixation, closed reduction). One of the most helpful pieces of information in this situation may be the patient's chart from the previous injury. If the patient has no history of trauma to the affected joint, further questioning should revolve around history of gout, infection, and RA. Exact symptomatology of the pain should be acquired, including when the pain started and when it occurs, if the pain gets worse on activity, if the pain is continuous, if the pain affects multiple joints on the ipsilateral side, and if the pain is bilateral.

Table 10-1

Helpful Hints

Differentiating Types of Arthritis

Post-Traumatic Arthritis	**Rheumatoid Arthritis**
History of trauma/surgery to affected joint	Family history of RA
No extra-articular symptoms	Extra-articular manifestations (rheumatoid nodules, fatigue, malaise)
Unilateral	Bilateral/symmetrical
Most common in tibiotalar/subtalar joints	Most common in MTP joints and forefoot.
Radiographs demonstrate joint space narrowing, subchondral sclerosis, and osteophyte formation	Radiographs demonstrate juxta-articular osteoporosis, subchondral cysts, and erosive changes

Examination

Physical exam of the arthritic foot and ankle (Table 10-2), unlike in acute injuries of the foot and ankle which preclude a complete exam due to patient pain/discomfort, should be performed to the fullest extent possible to create a baseline assessment of function. Two of the most fundamental aspects of the exam that should always be performed in a patient with suspected arthritis, no matter the etiology, are gait analysis and ranging of the joints.

Gait analysis begins prior to the patient taking a step, with analysis of abnormal wear on his or her shoes.[11] Standing foot and ankle alignment should be examined from behind to assess for varus/valgus deformities of the hindfoot. During the gait cycle, one should note any deviation in the hindfoot, and if any hammer or claw toe deformities are present.

Assessing functional range of motion (ROM) in the foot and ankle joints on the first visit can be helpful in assessing future progress or deterioration. Both passive and active ROM should be assessed bilaterally for comparison (see Table 10-2 for norms).

Table 10-2

Methods for Examining the Arthritic Foot and Ankle

Examination	*Technique*	*Illustration*	*Grading*			*Significance*
Range of motion	Examine active and passive range of motion					Determine extent of arthritic changes
			Joint	**Motion**	**Normal ROM**	
		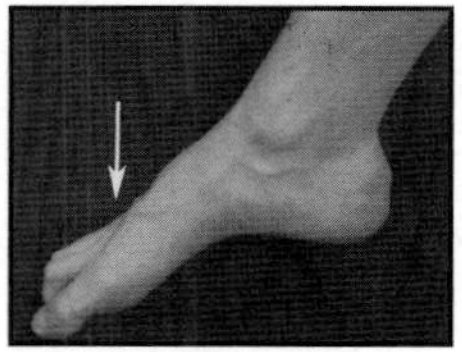	Tibiotalar	Ankle plantar flexion	0 to 50 degrees	
		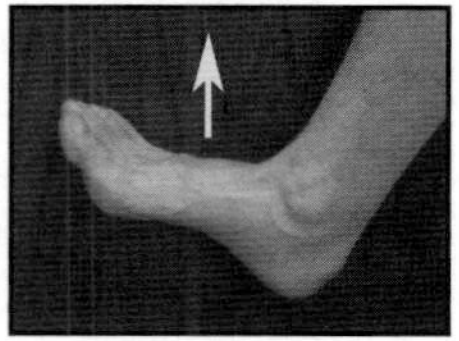		Ankle dorsi-flexion	0 to 20 degrees	

(continued)

Table 10-2 (continued)

METHODS FOR EXAMINING THE ARTHRITIC FOOT AND ANKLE

Examination	*Technique*	*Illustration*	*Grading*			*Significance*
Range of motion	Examine active and passive range of motion					Determine extent of arthritic changes
			JOINT	**MOTION**	**NORMAL ROM**	
		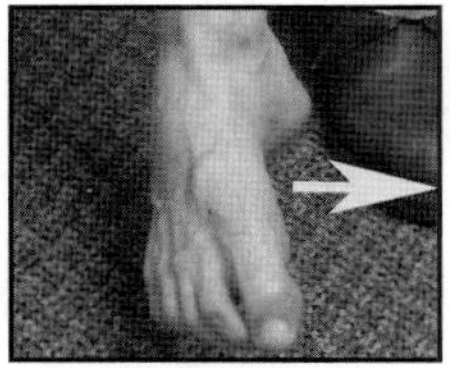	Subtalar	Foot inversion	0 to 35 degrees	
		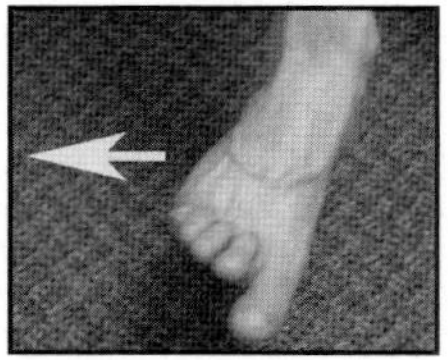		Foot eversion	0 to 25 degrees	

(continued)

Table 10-2 (continued)

Methods for Examining the Arthritic Foot and Ankle

Examination	*Technique*	*Illustration*	*Grading*			*Significance*
Range of motion	Examine active and passive range of motion					Determine extent of arthritic changes
			Joint	**Motion**	**Normal ROM**	
		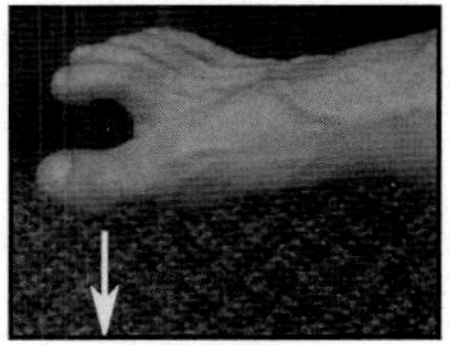	MTP	MTP flexion	0 to 30 degrees	
		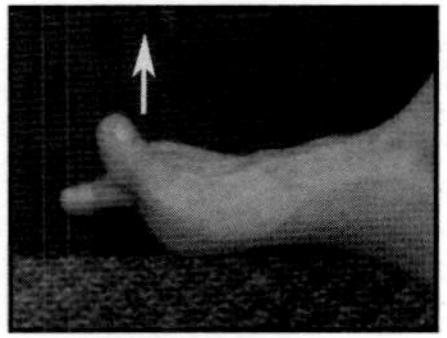		MTP extension	0 to 80 degrees	

(continued)

Table 10-2 (continued)

Methods for Examining the Arthritic Foot and Ankle

Examination	*Technique*	*Illustration*	*Grading*			*Significance*
Range of motion	Examine active and passive range of motion					Determine extent of arthritic changes
			Joint	**Motion**	**Normal ROM**	
			Interphalangeal (IP)	IP flexion	0 to 50 degrees	
				IP extension	0 to 80 degrees	
Strength	Manual strength testing of foot/ankle joints		Grade 5 = Full strength Grade 4 = <Full strength Grade 3 = Movement with gravity Grade 2 = Movement without gravity Grade 1 = Visible contraction			Determine any muscle/tendinous insufficiency or nerve injury

(continued)

Table 10-2 (continued)

Methods for Examining the Arthritic Foot and Ankle

Examination	*Technique*	*Illustration*	*Grading*	*Significance*
Gait analysis	Examine patient from behind and during normal gait cycles	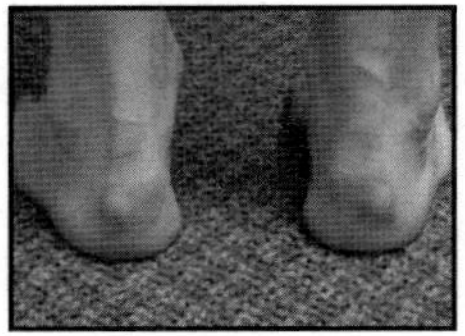		Determine valgus/varus deformities of the hindfoot
Sensory	Examine using a pinwheel or monofilament in dermatomal pattern distal to proximal			Determine if any nerve dysfunction exists in addition to arthritis (ie, Charcot's foot)

Pathoanatomy

The majority of this section will be used to discuss the pathoanatomy of post-traumatic ankle arthritis resulting from underlying abnormal ankle mechanics. Traumatic injuries of the ankle include fractures of the malleoli and associated ligamentous injury, fractures of the tibial plafond, and fractures of the talus. In all of these injuries, 2 of the most well-studied factors with strong correlations to the development of arthritis are inadequate reductions[3,14,15] and severity of injury to the articular cartilage.[3,16]

When discussing arthritis of the ankle, it is important to differentiate its pathophysiology from that of the hip and knee. Unlike the hip and knee joints, the ankle functions primarily as a rolling joint with congruent surfaces at high load, whereas the hip and knee function in a combination of rolling and rotating with noncongruent surfaces.[2,3] This combination of motions utilizing noncongruent surfaces may have a role in the development of osteoarthritis (OA) in the hip and knee, whereas the ankle's uniform rolling action and congruency protects it from primary OA but predisposes it to post-traumatic arthritis.[2,3]

A final concept relevant to the development of arthritis in the ankle is the unique properties of the articular cartilage. While the knee, for example, has varying thicknesses of cartilage (from 1 to 6 mm), ankle cartilage is relatively uniform in thickness, ranging from only 1 to 1.7 mm.[17-19] The thinner, more uniform cartilage in the ankle joint better equalizes stress over its congruent surface. Furthermore, compared to the articular cartilage of the hip and knee, ankle cartilage resists deterioration under normal physiological conditions, even into one's later years.[17-19]

With regard to the pathogenesis of RA, the characteristic progressive forefoot deformity begins with inflammation and proliferation of the MTP joint synovium, leading to distention of the capsule, loss of the stabilizing structures, and destruction of the articular cartilage. This loss of stability makes these structures extremely sensitive to deformity imposed by routine forces exerted on the foot. The dorsiflexion forces exerted on the MTP joints cause a progressive subluxation and

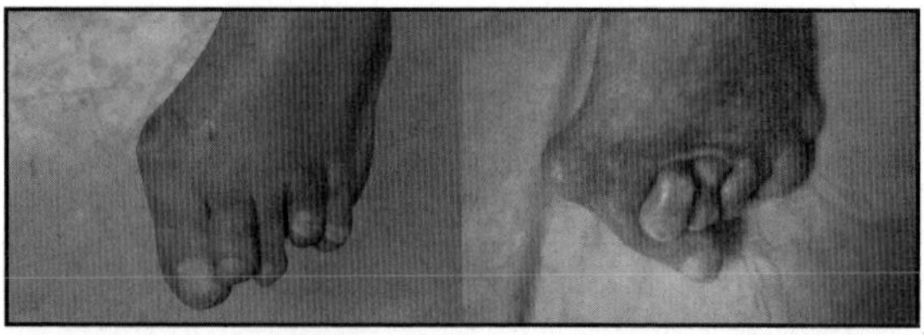

Figure 10-1. Examples of early and late forefoot RA.

eventual dorsal dislocation. As the proximal phalanx dislocates dorsally onto the neck of the metatarsal, the metatarsal head is forced plantar and the plantar fat pad pulled distal to the metatarsal heads. The resulting hammer toe and claw toe formation occurs because of an imbalance between the intrinsic and extrinsic muscles. The hallux undergoes a similar degeneration that most often drives it into valgus (Figure 10-1).[7, 20]

Imaging

When suspicious of arthritis in the foot and ankle, radiographic examination should include weight-bearing anteroposterior (AP), lateral, and medial oblique views of the foot and AP, lateral, and mortise views of the ankle. In the foot, both the talocalcaneal and talo-first metatarsal angles should be measured. In patients with post-traumatic arthritis, as in those with primary osteoarthritis, radiographic findings include joint space narrowing, subchondral sclerosis, and osteophyte formation (Figure 10-2). Bony findings unique to RA include juxta-articular osteoporosis and subcortical cysts (more than 3 with dull margins in an eccentric location are usually indicative of RA). In late disease, large erosions and bone destruction are seen, in addition to damage of the surrounding soft tissue structures. End-stage RA is noted by malalignment, displacement, and ankylosis of the joints.

In patients with suspected RA, in addition to the affected foot and ankle, the most commonly affected joints (the contralateral foot and ankle, hands, and C-spine) should be assessed for early disease. Two modalities often overlooked in the diagnosis of RA are ultrasound with high-resolution probes

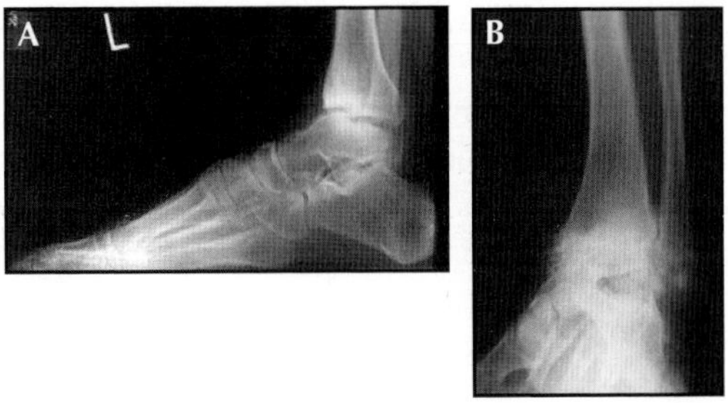

Figure 10-2. (A) AP and (B) lateral radiographs demonstrating post-traumatic arthritis of the ankle joint. Note the joint space narrowing, subchondral sclerosis, and osteophyte formation.

(7.5 MHz and greater) and magnetic resonance imaging (MRI).[20] Ultrasound can be used to quickly screen for superficial sites of inflammatory involvement, although clinical evidence of this in the literature is limited. MRI, though expensive, can best identify early stages of the disease, such as synovial hyperemia, synovitis, effusions, and bone marrow edema.[20]

TREATMENT

One of the important aspects concerning the treatment of foot and ankle arthritis is early recognition in order to prevent further deterioration of the affected joint. When a patient presents with foot and ankle arthritis, conservative therapy should first be attempted, using surgical intervention only if therapeutic options fail.

Conservative Treatment

Conservative treatment for foot and ankle arthritis is often indicated, although there is scant evidence for its ability to stave off further joint deterioration. Most protocols begin with a combination of pain relievers such as nonsteroidal anti-inflammatories, weight control, bracing, and footwear modification. This modified footwear might include a rigid insole and rocker-bottom sole, or a solid ankle cushion heel to help normalize gait pattern. The use of intra-articular corticosteroid injections is still controversial, with limited and temporary results at best. A trial period of immobilization in a plaster walking cast can simulate the feel of a fused ankle, since reducing ankle motion while walking helps to alleviate pain. In patients with RA, systemic drug therapy with one or a combination of the disease modifying antirheumatic drugs such as methotrexate, Remicade (infliximab), or Humira (adalimumab), would also be part of the treatment protocol.

Surgical Treatment

Operative Treatment for the Ankle

Operative treatment for tibiotalar arthritis is perhaps the most well-studied of all the joints in the foot and ankle. Surgical options range from arthroscopic surgical débridement to arthrodesis and arthroplasty. Arthroscopic surgical débridement is usually reserved for situations when only mild radiographic changes are noted and there are obvious impinging osteophytes, loose bodies, or isolated osteochondral lesions.

For advanced arthritis, marked joint-space narrowing, and varus/valgus deformities, one should consider either arthrodesis or arthroplasty. Arthrodesis has been the mainstay for end-stage ankle arthritis for over 50 years. Numerous techniques and approaches exist with a wide variety of stabilization techniques, which are beyond the scope of this chapter. The optimal position for ankle fusion has been well described, which is neutral dorsiflexion, 5 degrees of hindfoot valgus, and external rotation comparable to the contralateral limb. Unfortunately, ankle arthrodesis results in a 60% to 70% loss of sagittal motion, as well as decreased motion at the subtalar joint.[21] Clinically, walking speed is decreased by 16%, and an increased incidence of arthritis in joints of the hindfoot and midfoot has been observed, in addition to other complications (Figures 10-3 and 10-4).[22]

Ideally, one would prefer to maintain full ROM at the ankle joint, hence the increasing popularity of ankle arthroplasty over the past 5 to 10 years. First-generation designs proved to be unpopular because of extensive rates of loosening and osteolysis. Second-generation designs, although improving upon rates of osteolysis, had increased polyethylene wear and

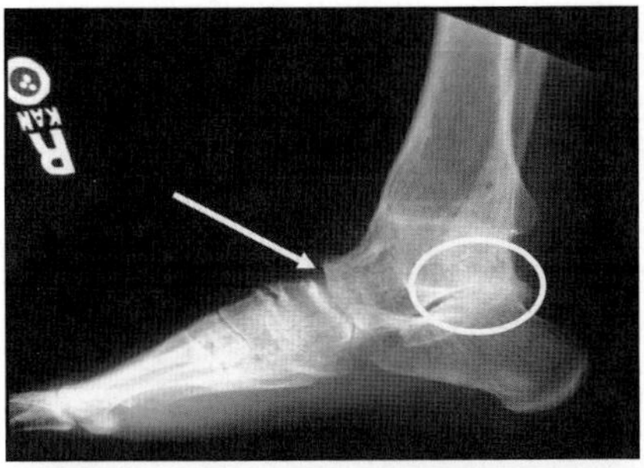

Figure 10-3. Lateral radiograph demonstrating degenerative changes in the talonavicular and subtalar joints following an ankle fusion.

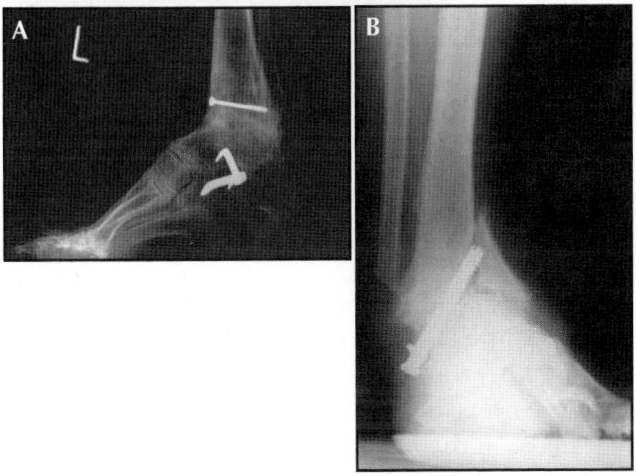

Figure 10-4. Radiographs demonstrating potential complications from failed ankle arthrodesis.

failure due to painful impingement, subluxation, or complete dislocation of components. All modern designs consist of 3 components: a metallic baseplate fixed to the tibia, a domed metallic component that resurfaces the talus, and a bearing surface made of ultra-high molecular weight polyethylene interposed between the tibial and talar components. Fixed-bearing systems lock the polyethylene component into the baseplate (Agility [Depuy, Warsaw, IN]) while mobile-bearing systems (Hintegra [Integra, Plainsboro, NJ], STAR [Small Bone Innovations, Inc, New York, NY], and Salto Talaris [Tornier, Inc., Edina, MN]) leave it free (Figure 10-5). Intermediate and long-term reports with modern systems have demonstrated improved outcomes with few complications compared to prior generations.[23] Presently, the indications for total ankle arthroplasty are limited and proper patient selection is

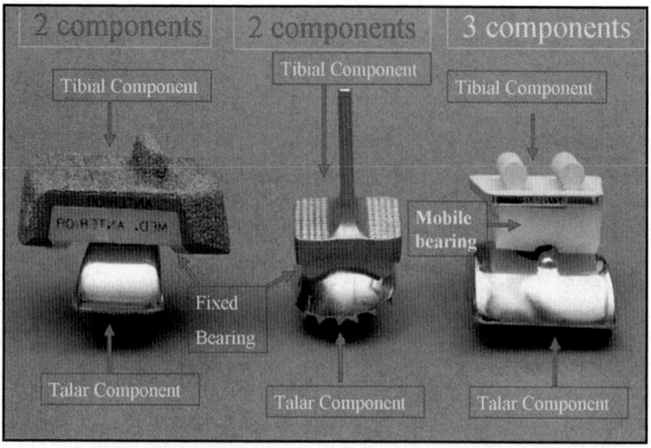

Figure 10-5. Note the differences between the older fixed-bearing ankle arthroplasty implants and current 3 component implant with a mobile bearing.

fundamental. The ideal patient is older than 50, weighing less than 200 pounds, with minimal deformity to the ankle joint. While currently not the most common treatment for ankle arthritis, ankle arthroplasty may become the treatment mainstay for this problem in the future.

Operative Treatment for the Midfoot and Hindfoot

Gold standard operative treatment of arthritis in both the midfoot and hindfoot involves arthrodesis of the involved joints. Because one of the primary concerns with arthrodesis is loss of motion, if the fourth and fifth tarsometatarsal joints are involved, the cuboid should not be fused to the lateral cuneiform in order to maintain flexibility.[7] Involvement of the 3 joints of the hindfoot (subtalar, talonavicular, and calcaneocuboid) is usually a late finding of RA, and involvement of all 3 joints is rare. Opinions vary widely on the number and combination of joints that should be fused in cases of isolated arthritis. For example, an advantage of isolated subtalar joint arthrodesis is preservation of motion of the transverse tarsal joint (Figure 10-6), but addition of the talonavicular and

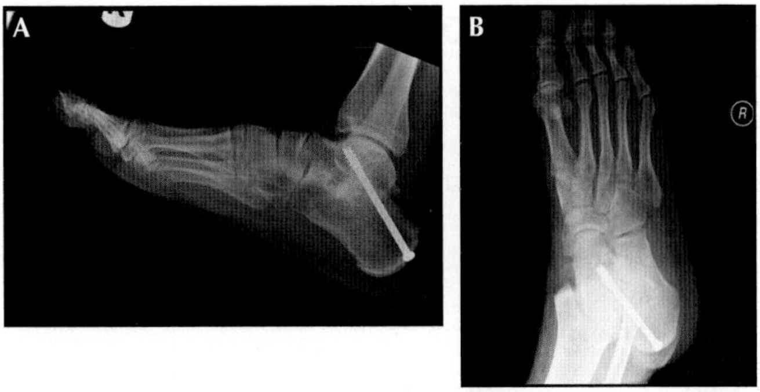

Figure 10-6. (A) Lateral and (B) oblique radiographs demonstrating successful subtalar arthrodesis.

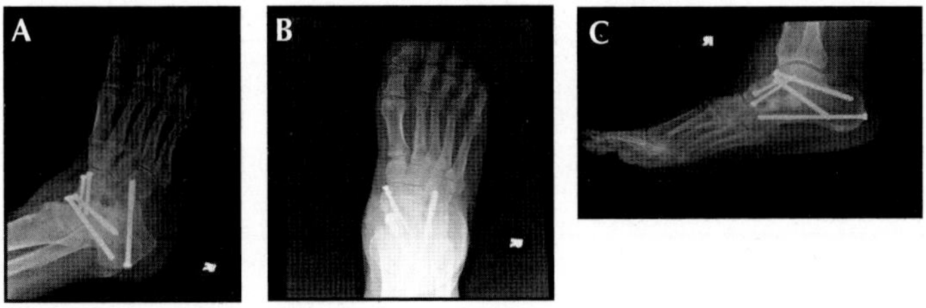

Figure 10-7. (A) AP, (B) lateral, and (C) oblique radiographs demonstrating successful triple arthrodesis.

calcaneocuboid joints add stability to the hindfoot. Triple arthrodesis is indicated when disease involves all 3 joints of the hindfoot (Figure 10-7). Positive results have been reported after triple arthrodesis with upward of 98% successful fusion rates.[7,24,25]

Operative Treatment for the Hallux

Arthrodesis of the first MTP joint is currently the most popular modality of treatment for hallux valgus due to arthritic changes. The arthrodesis provides stability to help protect the hallux and the lesser toes from future deforming forces. The recommended position of arthrodesis of the MTP joint is neutral rotation, 10 to 15 degrees of valgus, and 20 to 30 degrees of dorsiflexion in relation to the first metatarsal or 5 to 10 degrees in relation to the floor.[7]

Conclusion

Early diagnosis and recognition of foot and ankle arthritis is paramount in preventing long-term morbidity. Patients with risk factors such as prior trauma and family history of RA should be warned to keep a watchful eye on the development of symptoms so that intervention can proceed early in the disease process.

References

1. Cushnaghan J, Dieppe P. Study of 500 patients with limb joint osteoarthritis. I. Analysis by age, sex, and distribution of symptomatic joint sites. *Ann Rheum Dis.* 1991;50(1):8-13.
2. Huch K, Kuettner KE, Dieppe P. Osteoarthritis in ankle and knee joints. *Semin Arthritis Rheum.* 1997;26(4):667-674.
3. Thomas RH, Daniels TR. Ankle arthritis. *J Bone Joint Surg Am.* 2003;85-A(5):923-936.
4. Wilson MG, Michet CJ, Jr., Ilstrup DM, Melton LJ 3rd. Idiopathic symptomatic osteoarthritis of the hip and knee: a population-based incidence study. *Mayo Clin Proc.* 1990;65(9):1214-1221.
5. Valderrabano V, Horisberger M, Russell I, Dougall H, Hintermann B. Etiology of ankle osteoarthritis. *Clin Orthop Relat Res.* 2009;467(7): 1800-1806.
6. Fleming A, Crown JM, Corbett M. Early rheumatoid disease. I. Onset. *Ann Rheum Dis.* 1976;35(4):357-360.
7. Jaakkola JI, Mann RA. A review of rheumatoid arthritis affecting the foot and ankle. *Foot Ankle Int.* 2004;25(12):866-874.
8. Michelson J, Easley M, Wigley FM, Hellmann D. Foot and ankle problems in rheumatoid arthritis. *Foot Ankle Int.* 1994;15(11):608-613.
9. Turner DE, Helliwell PS, Emery P, Woodburn J. The impact of rheumatoid arthritis on foot function in the early stages of disease: a clinical case series. *BMC Musculoskelet Disord.* 2006;7:102.
10. Vainio K. The rheumatoid foot; a clinical study with pathological and roentgenological comments. *Ann Chir Gynaecol Fenn Suppl.* 1956;45(1):1-107.
11. van der Leeden M, Steultjens MP, Terwee CB, et al. A systematic review of instruments measuring foot function, foot pain, and foot-related disability in patients with rheumatoid arthritis. *Arthritis Rheum.* 2008;59(9):1257-1269.
12. van der Leeden M, Steultjens MP, Ursum J, et al. Prevalence and course of forefoot impairments and walking disability in the first eight years of rheumatoid arthritis. *Arthritis Rheum.* 2008;59(11):1596-1602.
13. Vidigal E, Jacoby RK, Dixon AS, Ratliff AH, Kirkup J. The foot in chronic rheumatoid arthritis. *Ann Rheum Dis.* 1975;34(4):292-297.

14. Macko VW, Matthews LS, Zwirkoski P, Goldstein SA. The joint-contact area of the ankle. The contribution of the posterior malleolus. *J Bone Joint Surg Am.* 1991;73(3):347-351.
15. Rüedi T. Fractures of the lower end of the tibia into the ankle joint: results 9 years after open reduction and internal fixation. *Injury.* 1973;5(2):130-134.
16. Marsh JL, Buckwalter J, Gelberman R, et al. Articular fractures: does an anatomic reduction really change the result? *J Bone Joint Surg Am.* 2002;84-A(7):1259-1271.
17. Ateshian GA, Soslowsky LJ, Mow VC. Quantitation of articular surface topography and cartilage thickness in knee joints using stereophotogrammetry. *J Biomech.* 1991;24(8):761-776.
18. Athanasiou KA, Niederauer GG, Schenck RC, Jr. Biomechanical topography of human ankle cartilage. *Ann Biomed Eng.* 1995;23(5):697-704.
19. Shepherd DE, Seedhom BB. Thickness of human articular cartilage in joints of the lower limb. *Ann Rheum Dis.* 1999;58(1):27-34.
20. Sommer OJ, Kladosek A, Weiler V, Czembirek H, Boeck M, Stiskal M. Rheumatoid arthritis: a practical guide to state-of-the-art imaging, image interpretation, and clinical implications. *Radiographics.* 2005;25(2):381-398.
21. Hintermann B, Nigg BM. Influence of arthrodeses on kinematics of the axially loaded ankle complex during dorsiflexion/plantarflexion. *Foot Ankle Int.* 1995;16(10):633-636.
22. Coester LM, Saltzman CL, Leupold J, Pontarelli W. Long-term results following ankle arthrodesis for post-traumatic arthritis. *J Bone Joint Surg Am.* 2001;83-A(2):219-228.
23. Guyer AJ, Richardson G. Current concepts review: total ankle arthroplasty. *Foot Ankle Int.* 2008;29(2):256-264.
24. Figgie MP, O'Malley MJ, Ranawat C, Inglis AE, Sculco TP. Triple arthrodesis in rheumatoid arthritis. *Clin Orthop Relat Res.* 1993(292):250-254.
25. Pell RF 4th, Myerson MS, Schon LC. Clinical outcome after primary triple arthrodesis. *J Bone Joint Surg Am.* 2000;82(1):47-57.

11

Plantar Fasciitis and Plantar Heel Pain

Premjit S. Deol, DO and Terrence M. Philbin, DO

Introduction

Plantar heel pain can often be the bane of the orthopedist or primary care physician. This is often due to a relatively poor understanding of this region of the foot. The proximity of numerous anatomic structures within this small area often creates ambiguity in formulating a diagnosis for heel pain. A thorough knowledge of topographical anatomy of the calcaneus and the complex relationship of the plantar heel structures are critical to establishing a diagnosis. The burden, therefore, falls upon the physician to clearly identify the underlying etiology in order to appropriately treat the patient and return him or her to a full and active lifestyle.

Hurwitz SR, Parekh SG. *Musculoskeletal Examination of the Foot and Ankle: Making the Complex Simple* (pp. 196-213).

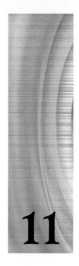

Plantar heel pain can have debilitating effects upon athletes and nonathletes alike. Proximal plantar fasciitis represents the most common cause, afflicting approximately 80% of patients presenting with plantar heel pain.[1] It has been reported to afflict approximately 2 million people annually,[2] with an occurrence rate of over 10% in runners.[3] With the national annual costs for the treatment of plantar heel pain in the millions of dollars, treatment strategies are continually being developed to avert the onset and decrease the duration of symptoms.

History

The first modern published description of plantar heel pain was by Wood in 1812, when he suspected it was related to an infection of the plantar fascia.[4] Continued investigation into the role of the plantar fascia in patients with heel pain led to increased understanding of its biomechanical contributions. The plantar fascia has been shown to contribute to numerous components of stance and gait, including support of weight bearing, propulsion, shock absorption, and adaptation to uneven ground.[5]

In 1954, Hicks suggested the foot and heel have a unique anatomic relationship between the bony and soft tissue elements by which mechanical work was able to be achieved for gait.[6] This relationship was described as that of an arch-like truss formed from the osseous architecture of the calcaneus, midtarsal joints, and metatarsals. The plantar fascia, through its attachments to the calcaneus and each of the proximal phalanxes, acts as a tie rod connecting each end of the truss. During the propulsive phase of gait, dorsiflexion of the metatarsophalangeal (MTP) joints places tension across the plantar fascia as it traverses underneath the metatarsal heads. This shortening of the fascia elevates the arch of the midfoot through the pull of the tie rod on the overlying truss. This phenomenon has come to be known as the *windlass mechanism*.

Within the context of this biomechanical framework, additional anatomic structures within the heel may be underappreciated in their potential contribution to plantar heel pain. Baxter was credited with eliciting the role of entrapment

Table 11-1

ADDITIONAL DIFFERENTIAL DIAGNOSES FOR PLANTAR HEEL PAIN

Calcaneal stress fracture or bony contusion	Infection/abscess
Complete rupture of plantar fascia	Peripheral neuropathy/ radiculopathy
Posterior tibial tendinitis	Degenerative arthrosis of adjacent joints
Flexor hallucis longus tendinitis	Inflammatory arthropathy
Tumor (bony or soft tissue)	Lower extremity malalignment

neuropathies as a potential source of heel pain in those recalcitrant to treatment for plantar fasciitis.[7] Plantar fat pad atrophy, tarsal tunnel syndrome, midsubstance plantar fasciitis, and various other causes of heel pain must also be contemplated when assessing patients presenting with complaints of plantar heel pain (Table 11-1).

EXAMINATION

A systematic approach is crucial in the evaluation of heel pain. An anatomic assessment from proximal to distal can facilitate examination of all bony and soft tissue structures within the heel (Figure 11-1). The anatomic complexity surrounding the os calcis is simplified by assessing each of its major components, beginning with the posterior tuberosity. Posterior heel pain originating from insertional Achilles tendinosis may result in hypertrophy around the posterior tubercle. Fascial extension from the Achilles tendon insertion continues in part around the calcaneus to blend with fibers of the plantar fascia.[8] Contracture within the Achilles tendon may contribute to increased tension within the plantar tissues of the foot, creating increased stress and plantar pain.[9] The

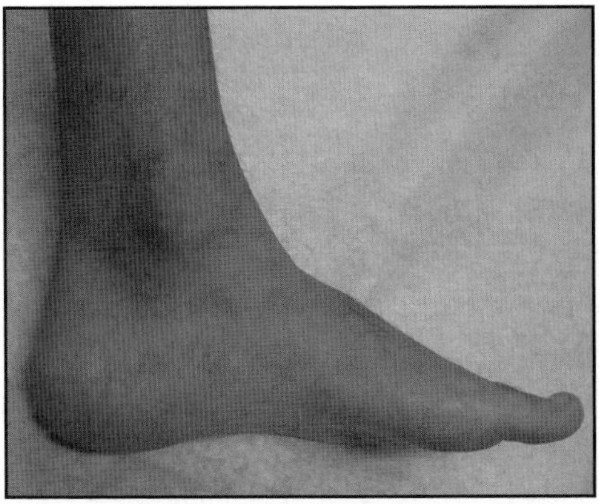

Figure 11-1. Topography of the foot and heel. Assessment of patients with heel pain should be conducted in a systematic fashion. Proceeding from proximal anatomy distally ensures a thorough review of all anatomic structures. Evaluation must include not only all bony and soft tissue elements, but underlying neurovascular structures as well.

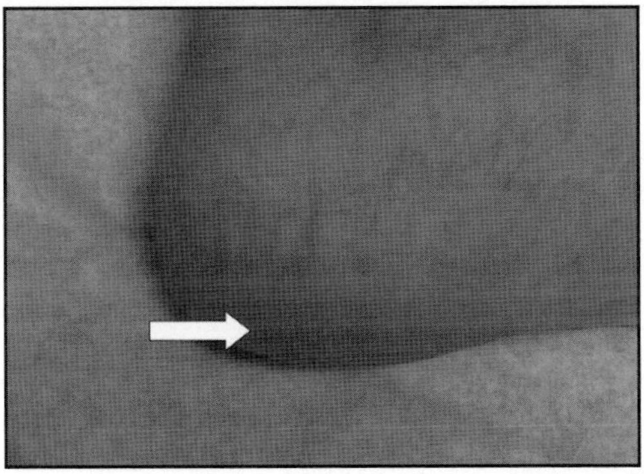

Figure 11-2. Calcaneal fat pad. The plantar fat pad is located beneath the calcaneal tuberosity (white arrow). Adjacent fascial attachments provide stability to the fat pad, aiding in shock absorption during weight bearing. Pain localized to the direct plantar aspect of the calcaneal tuberosity in an older population may represent atrophy of this structure. Instability of the fat pad due to fascial disruption is diagnosed with increased mobility of the plantar soft tissues beneath the tuberosity.

calcaneal fat pad is positioned on the plantar aspect of the calcaneus (Figure 11-2). Atrophy, incompetence, or instability of this structure places an increased load upon the calcaneus during weight bearing, creating repetitive microtrauma and

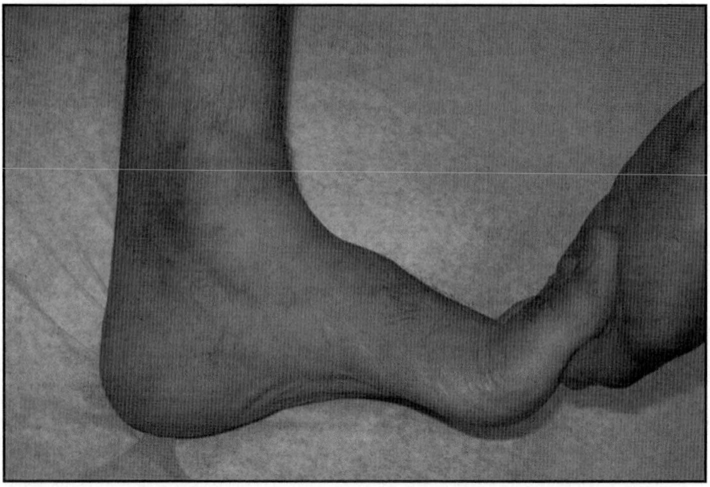

Figure 11-3. Windlass mechanism. The plantar fascia extends from the plantar aspect of the medial calcaneal tuberosity to each of the toes, inserting distal to the MTP joints. The toes extend during the propulsive phase of gait, creating tension across the plantar fascia. This acts to functionally raise the arch of the midfoot. Replication of this phenomenon with direct palpation over the plantar fascia during physical examination will replicate the pain associated with plantar fasciitis.

a potential source of pain.[8,10] In rare cases, this may lead to the development of a stress reaction within the calcaneus. Coronally directed compression of the calcaneus will replicate the patient's pain in the scenario of calcaneal stress fractures.

The medial and lateral plantar tuberosities of the calcaneus are distal to the fat pad. The central band of the plantar fascia extends from the medial tuberosity to each of the toes. Its insertion on the anteromedial aspect of the medial calcaneal tuberosity is the most common site of maximal tenderness in insertional plantar fasciitis.[11] This major band is flanked by secondary medial and lateral bands, covering the abductor hallucis and inserting into the base of the fifth metatarsal, respectively. Passive dorsiflexion of the toes with the ankle dorsiflexed engages the windlass mechanism and typically exacerbates the symptoms of plantar fasciitis[12] (Figure 11-3). Less commonly, midsubstance plantar fascia pain is the result of repetitive microtrauma to the plantar fascia. In rare circumstances, an ultimate tensile failure of the plantar fascia can result in a complete rupture with a palpable loss of the longitudinal fibers across the plantar aspect of the foot.

Compressive neuropathies can often mimic or contribute to the pain of plantar fasciitis and must be ruled out. As the posterior tibial nerve crosses beneath the flexor retinaculum along the medial aspect of the calcaneus, entrapment may result in tarsal tunnel syndrome. Provocative percussion testing along the course of the tarsal tunnel reproducing radicular symptoms is indicative of local compression (Figure 11-4). One of the more commonly overlooked sources of heel pain is due to compression of the first branch of the lateral plantar nerve, also known as Baxter's nerve. Its innervation to the periosteum of the medial calcaneal tuberosity, abductor digiti quinti, and flexor brevis muscles can be misinterpreted as pain originating from the plantar fascia. The key differentiating component is tenderness along the medial aspect of the hindfoot distal to the flexor retinaculum, between the deep fascia of the abductor hallucis and medial-caudal margin of the medial head of the quadrates plantae. Helpful hints and methods for examination for plantar heel pain may be found in Tables 11-2 and 11-3.

PATHOANATOMY

The particular mechanism for the pathogenesis for heel pain is linked to the underlying etiology. As a particular anatomic structure is placed under increased mechanical stresses surpassing its normal threshold, an inflammatory response is generated in an effort to stimulate healing. If the stresses are continually greater than what these structures are able to tolerate, the cumulative microtrauma compromises the body's repair efforts, leading to a pattern of chronic inflammation. The biomechanics of the lower extremity and foot position greatly impact the stresses on the plantar structures and fascia. Tightness within the lower extremity has been noted to alter the gait cycle, thereby overloading the foot and risking injury through repetitive microtrauma.[13] Over-pronators typically have a highly mobile foot, leading to tissue elongation from increased tension on the musculofascial structures.[14] In contrast, higher-arched feet often lack some of the necessary mobility needed to dissipate peak forces with loading, thereby

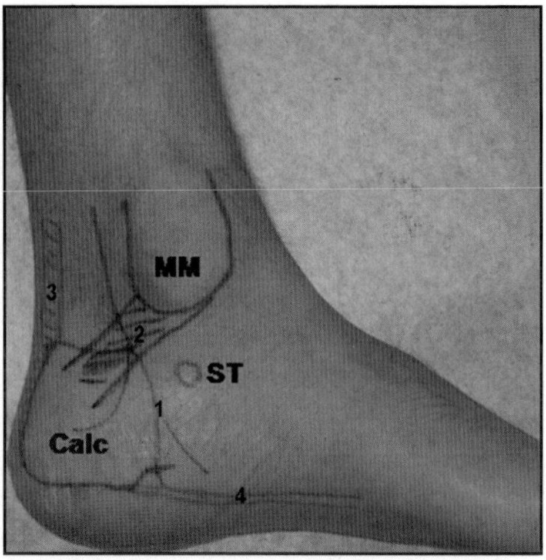

Figure 11-4A. Anatomic structures related to heel pain. (A) The examination of patients with heel pain begins with the primary osseous structures of the ankle and hindfoot, the medial malleolus and calcaneus. The tibial nerve (1) travels beneath the tarsal tunnel (2), which lies posterior to the sustentacular tali. The Achilles tendon (3) and plantar fascia (4) attachments can be directly palpated.

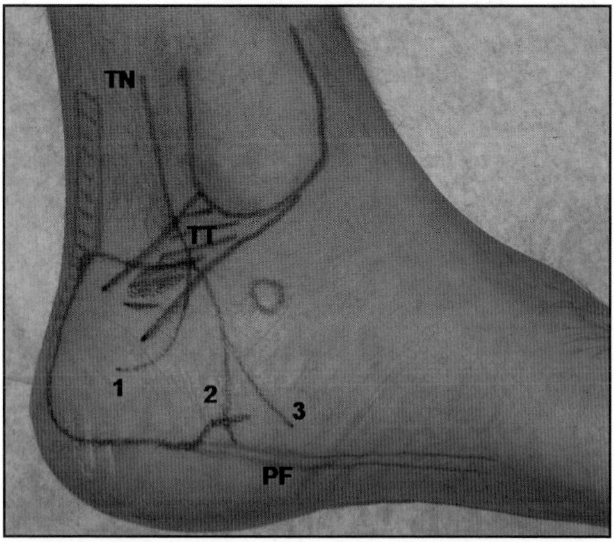

Figure 11-4B. The plantar fascia (PF) originates from the plantar aspect of the medial tuberosity of the calcaneus, extending longitudinally along the plantar aspect of the foot. The tibial nerve travels beneath the lucinate ligament of the flexor retinaculum, creating the tarsal tunnel. Its branches include (1) the calcaneal branch. (2) the lateral plantar nerve and (3) the medial plantar nerve. A compressive neuropathy of the lateral plantar nerve can occur as it travels along the insertion of the plantar fascia.

Table 11-2

HELPFUL HINTS FOR PLANTAR HEEL PAIN

Calcaneal stress fracture	Pain increases with activity/end up pain Positive squeeze test Positive MRI changes and occasionally on the x-ray
Tarsal tunnel	Burning pain Positive Tinel's test Electromyography (EMG) may be positive
Plantar fasciitis	Pain at the beginning of an activity/start up pain Pain over the medial insertion

Table 11-3

METHODS OF EXAMINATION

Calcaneal stress fracture	Positive squeeze test. Cup your hands around the heel and push side to side.
Tarsal tunnel	Positive Tine's test. Pain while tapping over the tarsal tunnel.
Plantar fasciitis	Pain over the medial insertion point. X marks the spot.

increasing the stresses transmitted with weight bearing to these same structures.[15]

Along the plantar aspect of the heel, atrophy of the fat pad begins after 40 years.[16] A gradual age-related loss of collagen, water, elastic fibers, and overall volume of the fat pad is attributed to creating a softer and thinner pad less equipped to dissipate load-bearing forces.[17] Forces across this region are transmitted through the plantar fascia along the medial longitudinal arch. As the plantar fascia experiences increased stress, microtears can develop and lead to collagen necrosis, angiofibroblastic hyperplasia, and chronic inflammation.[18] In accordance with Wolff's law, a secondary calcaneal traction spur may develop off the medial tuberosity. The location and direction of the traction spur can be variable but predominantly occurs at the origin of the flexor digitorum brevis.[19,20] This spur has been shown to lie directly along the primary lines of stress on the calcaneus.[21] The pain associated with plantar fasciitis is considered to be due to the increased strain within the soft tissue structures and not directly related to the presence of the resulting spur.

Compression of the posterior tibial nerve is commonly the result of a space-occupying lesion within the flexor retinaculum. Varicosities, bony spurs, adhesions, or soft tissue masses are the most commonly encountered.[16] Excessive pronation or hindfoot valgus may create a mechanical traction neuropathy, producing the symptoms of tarsal tunnel syndrome. Entrapment of the first branch of the lateral plantar nerve (LPN) predictably occurs as the nerve abruptly changes orientation from vertical to horizontal along the medial plantar heel.[22,23] Tethering of the nerve is created from the narrow, thickened fascial window created between the abductor hallucis and quadrates plantae. This is exacerbated in athletes who routinely balance upon their toes or compete in an en pointe position leading to abductor hallucis hypertrophy.[16,24] Less commonly, this branch of the LPN will be encroached upon by a calcaneal traction spur as it courses distal to the medial tuberosity.

Imaging

The diagnoses related to plantar heel pain can reliably be made based upon accurate and detailed review of the patient's history and clinical examination. The use of radiological investigation is used to support the clinical diagnosis and exclude less likely diagnoses. Routine weight-bearing radiographs of the foot and ankle can provide additional insight into overall alignment, skeletal architecture or presence of adjacent degenerative joint disease (Figure 11-5). The presence of a calcaneal traction spur or calcification within the plantar fascia may be identified incidentally and represent a secondary response to the increased soft tissue stresses (Figure 11-6). It has been reported that 50% of patients with plantar heel pain will not have evidence of a calcaneal traction spur.[16] Rarely does the

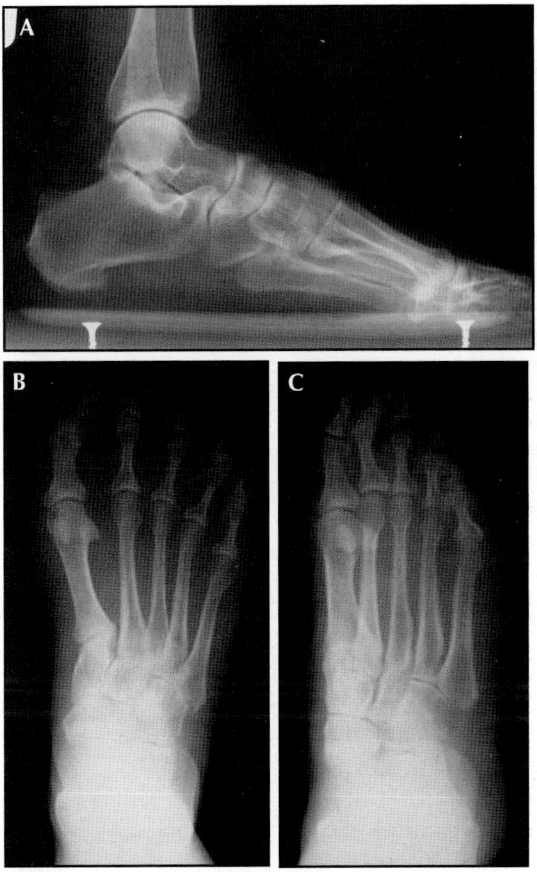

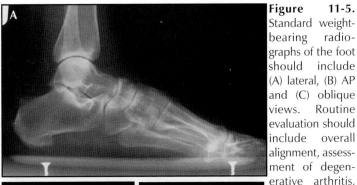

Figure 11-5. Standard weight-bearing radiographs of the foot should include (A) lateral, (B) AP and (C) oblique views. Routine evaluation should include overall alignment, assessment of degenerative arthritis, calcific tendinopathy and the exclusion of additional sources of pain.

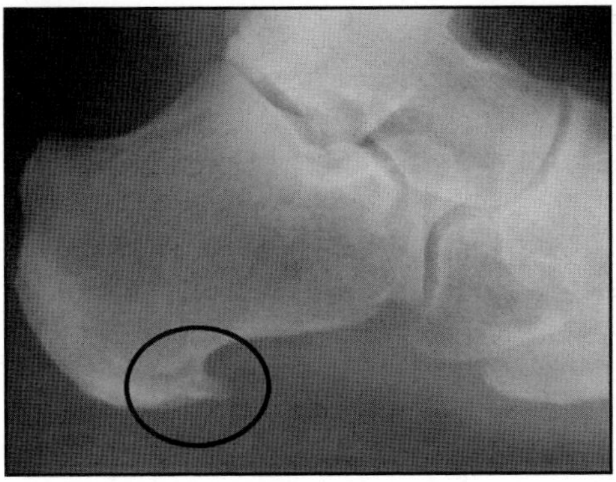

Figure 11-6. Calcaneal traction spur. Standard weight-bearing lateral radiographs of the foot often show evidence of underlying pathology. The presence of calcification along the insertion of the plantar fascia represents a secondary response to chronic traction stress on the periosteum of the calcaneus.

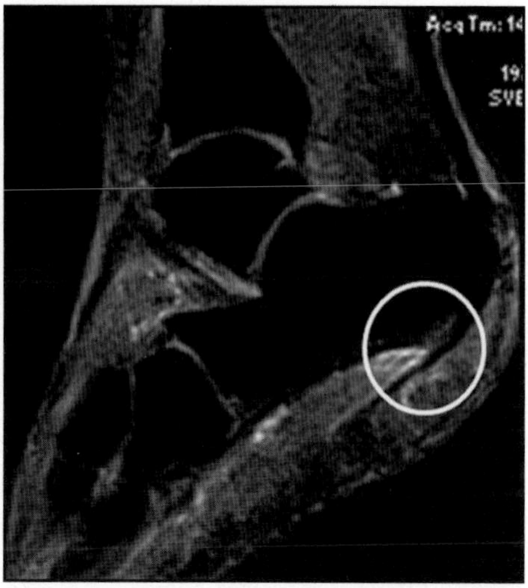

Figure 11-7. MRI sagittal view of plantar fasciitis. Evaluation of plantar heel pain with MRI may reveal additional pathology within the foot. The presence of bony edema related to repetitive stresses exerted at the insertion of the plantar fascia is visualized (white circle). Edema within the adjacent soft tissues and heel pad, along the course of the calcaneal traction spur, is compatible with the diagnosis of proximal plantar fasciitis.

radiographic evaluation alter the diagnosis or treatment algorithm based on the results of the history and physical exam findings.

Magnetic resonance imaging (MRI) of the foot and ankle is often utilized to evaluate the soft tissue components of the hindfoot in the presence of plantar heel pain. This can provide the practitioner with a greater appreciation for all contributing factors, in addition to establishing a context with which to discuss likely outcomes or prognosis. MRI is able to establish the extent of degenerative tendinosis or fasciitis, presence of space-occupying lesions in the context of compressive neuropathy, evaluate soft tissue masses, and assess for stress fractures or osteochondral injuries (Figures 11-7, 11-8, and 11-9). The use of triple-phase bone scans may help to distinguish between pain originating from skeletal components and soft tissue structures within the heel. Ultrasound has also been advocated as a more efficient and economical method by which to assess hypertrophy of the plantar fascia and compressibility of the heel fat pad.[20]

In the work-up of neurologic etiologies for heel pain, EMG and nerve conduction velocity studies are used to differentiate central from peripheral entrapment. The presence of proximal nerve impingement, or even a double-crush phenomenon, will

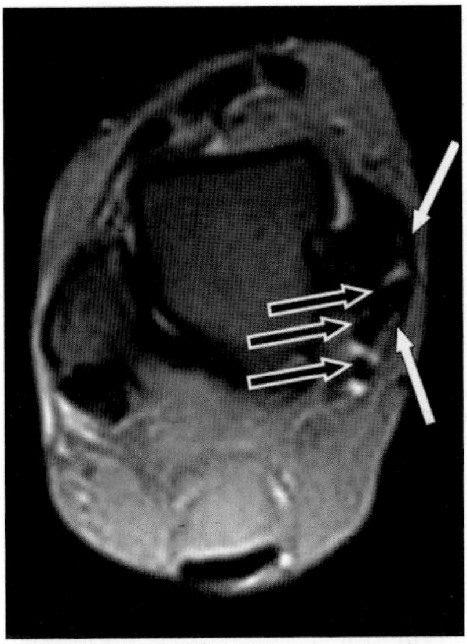

Figure 11-8. MRI axial view of contents within the tarsal tunnel. Evaluation of heel pain must also include evaluation of the tarsal tunnel. Compressive neuropathy of the tibial nerve at the level of the tarsal tunnel may mimic symptoms of plantar heel pain. The lucinate ligament (white arrows) extends from the medial malleolus to the medial wall of the calcaneus. Its contents include the major flexor tendons of the foot and the posterior tibial neurovascular bundle (black arrows).

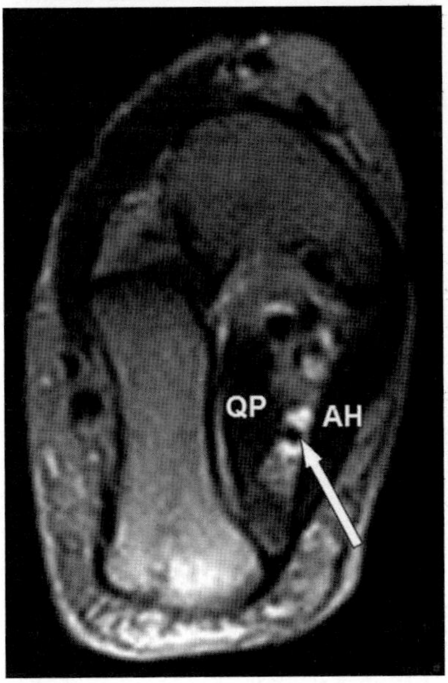

Figure 11-9. MRI axial view of lateral plantar nerve. The LPN (white arrow) descends into the plantar aspect of the foot as a branch of the posterior tibial nerve. As it courses along the medial aspect of the foot, it abruptly changes from a vertical to horizontal orientation. This occurs between the abductor hallucis and quadratus plantae muscles. Compression of the LPN in this region can produce pain referred to the heel.

greatly influence the prognosis related to peripheral nerve decompression. These studies can help to distinguish more subtle clinical presentations of peripheral nerve entrapment.

Treatment

Most patients that present to their physician's office for evaluation of plantar heel pain have dealt with symptoms for an extended period of time preceding their visit. The natural history of heel pain is favorable, as the majority of patients experience resolution of their pain without surgery. The frustration is that this can often take 6 months, even up to 1 year, to occur. A repetitive cycle of mild discomfort with periodic exacerbation of symptoms is not uncommon. A multimodal therapeutic approach is most successful in altering the natural history of the disease process. Routine management begins with conservative measures, which most commonly combines a stretching program with orthotics. Tissue-specific stretching of the plantar fascia has been shown to reliably alleviate the pain associated with plantar fasciitis and heel pain.[25] The use of orthotics allows for balancing of the foot and a redistribution of weight-bearing forces away from the heel. A multicenter investigation demonstrated significant improvement in outcomes for plantar fasciitis using over-the-counter inserts when combined with a stretching regimen.[2] The incorporation of anti-inflammatory medications, injections, night splints, or appropriate shoe wear to routine stretching and orthotics can produce a relatively high success rate in appropriate patients. In cases unresponsive to a combination of these measures, immobilization in a non–weight-bearing cast or boot may allow the time necessary to offload the plantar tissues to mount an adequate healing response. The use of extracorporeal shock wave therapy with electrohydraulic (high-energy) or electromagnetic (low-energy) devices has been shown to have good moderate-term success for chronic plantar fasciitis.[26,27] Unfortunately, the lack of insurance coverage for this noninvasive procedure has led to its fall from favor with many patients and practitioners. For those who have made good faith efforts at conservative care, several surgical options are available. Historically, the success rate of surgical intervention

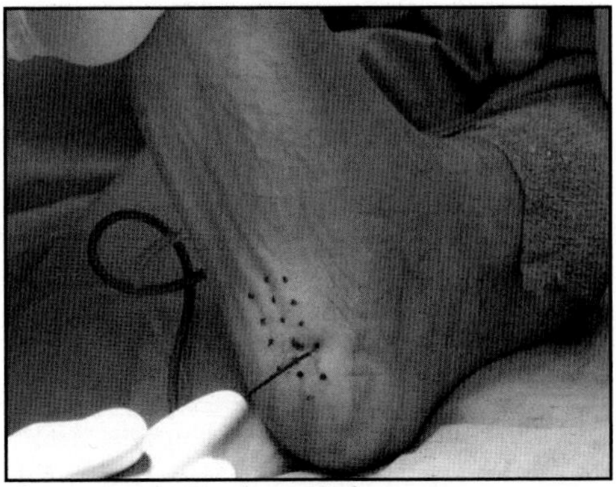

Figure 11-10. Bipolar radiofrequency treatment of the plantar fascia. In cases of recalcitrant plantar fasciitis, surgical intervention can often hasten recovery. Bipolar radiofrequency is a newer technology utilized in the surgical treatment of plantar fasciitis. Through an open or percutaneous (as shown) approach, a plasma field is generated by the device within the local tissues, which can induce an angiogenic response within the plantar fascia.

has fallen short of expectations, leading most physicians to exhaust conservative measures until the patient is unable to continue in his or her current state. In the athletic population, it is critical to be selective in both surgical dissection and in the release of anatomic structures to allow for a more expeditious recovery and return to sport.[28] The use of selective diagnostic anesthetic injections can be helpful to differentiate between multiple potential sources of heel pain. Bipolar radiofrequency technology has recently been advocated as a less invasive form of intervention for plantar fasciitis. Through either a percutaneous or limited open approach, it has been purported to abruptly interrupt the pain pathway and accentuate healing by stimulating an angiogenic response within the local hypovascular tissue, leading to a hastened recovery[29,39] (Figure 11-10). Although early results are promising, this technology has yet to withstand the scrutiny of prospective, longer-term follow up.

The surgical approach for plantar heel pain typically occurs from the medial aspect with a single oblique incision along the hindfoot. All attempts should be made to avoid incisions on the plantar aspect of the foot due to the high tension forces and a risk of wound complications. The advantage of the oblique medially based approach is accessibility to most of the anatomic structures of concern with plantar heel pain (Figure 11-11A). Decompression of the tarsal tunnel and the overlying flexor retinaculum are possible at the most proximal extent of the incision. Release of the fascia around the abductor hallucis and excision of any space occupying lesions, including varicosities, when engulfing the nerve are critical (Figure 11-11B). The first branch of the lateral plantar nerve can be traced between the abductor hallucis/quadrates plantae interval along the plantar calcaneus, utilizing a hemostat to release adhesions and assess for areas of impingement. In select cases, a decompression of the calcaneal spur or partial release of the plantar fascia of up to 40% is necessary.[31] A complete release of the plantar fascia is not advised as it can destabilize the windlass mechanism and radically change the biomechanics and stability of the foot. Complete plantar fascial release has been reported to result in stress fractures, vague lateral column pain, and stress fractures of the calcaneus and cuboid.[32]

Conclusion

The occurrence of plantar heel pain commonly signifies a short-lived hindrance for most patients. With a success rate of 85% to 95% when treated early with conservative measures, practitioners should have great optimism in returning athletes and the general population back to their routine activities.[1] For those without resolution of their pain, a distinction must be made between those with cases resistant to conservative measures from those with potentially incorrect working diagnoses. Those in need of surgical intervention will be greatly served by an accurate diagnosis related to specific pathology, allowing more selective decompressions and a faster recovery. A return to full activity can reliably be expected by 4 months following adequate physical therapy and sport specific conditioning. Although, patients should be cautioned that complete recovery may take up to a period of 1 year.

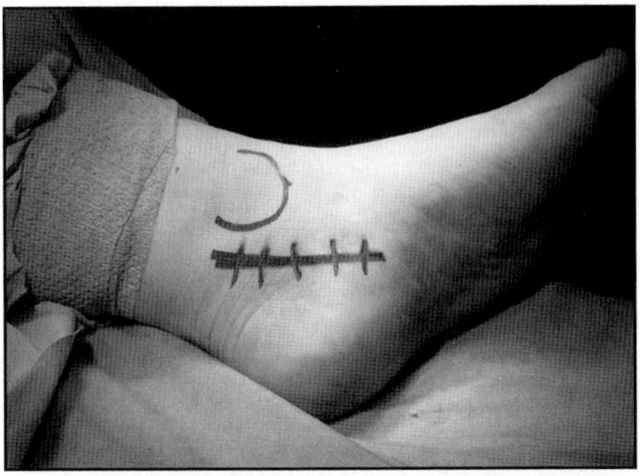

Figure 11-11A. Incision marked for open release of the tarsal tunnel and partial release of the medial portion of the plantar fascia.

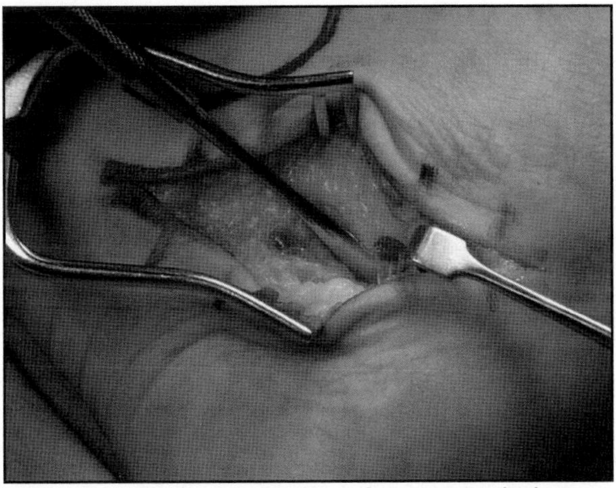

Figure 11-11B. Decompression of posterior tibial nerve with release of overlying fascia of the abductor. The surgical approach to plantar heel pain is from the medial aspect of the hindfoot. The oblique incision is based proximally at the level of the lucinate ligament and extends distally toward the insertion of the plantar fascia. This utilitarian incision allows for decompression of the posterior tibial nerve, release of the lateral plantar nerve and its branches, and partial release of the plantar fascia.

References

1. Tisdel CL. Heel pain. In: Richardson EG, ed. *Orthopedic Knowledge Update: Foot and Ankle*. 3rd ed. Rosemont, IL: AAOS; 2004:113-119.
2. Pfeffer GB, Bacchetti P, Deland J, et al. Comparison of custom and prefabricated orthoses in the initial treatment of proximal plantar fasciitis. *Foot Ankle Int*. 1999;20(4):214-221.
3. Chandler TJ, Kibler WB. A biomechanical approach to the prevention, treatment and rehabilitation of plantar fasciitis. *Sports Med*. 1993;15(5):344-352.
4. Lee TH, Maurus PB. Plantar heel pain. In: Coughlin MJ, Mann RA, Saltzman CL, eds. *Surgery of the Foot and Ankle*. 8th ed. Philadelphia, PA: Mosby Elsevier; 2007:689-705.
5. Norkin CC, Levangie PK. *Joint Structure and Function: A Comprehensive Analysis*. 4th ed. Philadelphia, PA: FA Davis; 2001.
6. Hicks JH. The mechanics of the foot. II. The plantar aponeurosis and the arch. *J Anat*.1954;88(1):25-30.
7. Baxter DE, Thigpen CM. Heel pain–operative results. *Foot Ankle*. 1984;5(1):16-25.
8. Snow SW, Bohne WH, DiCarlo E, Chang VK. Anatomy of the Achilles tendon and plantar fascia in relation to the calcaneus in various age groups. *Foot Ankle Int*. 1995;16(7):418-421.
9. Cheung JT, Zhang M, An KN. Effect of Achilles tendon loading on plantar fascia tension in the standing foot. *Clin Biomech (Bristol, Avon)*. 2006;21(2):194-203.
10. Buschmann WR, Jahss MH, Kummer F, Desai P, Gee RO, Ricci JL. Histology and histomorphometric analysis of the normal and atrophic heel fat pad. *Foot Ankle Int*. 1995;16(5):254-258.
11. Schon LC, Gruber F, Pfeffer GB. Plantar heel pain. In: Porter DA, Schon LC, eds. *Baxter's: The Foot and Ankle in Sports*. 2nd ed. Philadelphia, PA: Mosby; 2008: 226-239.
12. Carlson RE, Fleming LL, Hutton WC. The biomechanical relationship between the tendoachilles, plantar fascia and metatarsophalangeal joint dorsiflexion angle. *Foot Ankle Int*. 2000;21(1):18-25.
13. Harty J, Soffe K, O'Toole G, Stephens MM. The role of hamstring tightness in plantar fasciitis. *Foot Ankle Int*. 2005;26(12):1089-1092.
14. Bolgla LA, Malone TR. Plantar fasciitis and the windlass mechanism: a biomechanical link to clinical practice. *J Athle Train*. 2004;39(1):77-82.
15. Nachbauer W, Nigg BM. Effects of arch height of the foot on ground reaction forces in running. *Med Sci Sports Exerc*. 1992;24(11):1264-1269.
16. Pfeffer GB. Plantar heel pain. *Instr Course Lect*. 2001;50:521-531.
17. Ozdemir H, Soyuncu Y, Ozgorgen M, Dabak K. Effects of changes in heel fat pad thickness and elasticity on heel pain. *J Am Podiatr Med Assoc*. 2004;94(1):47-52.
18. Snider MP, Clancy WG, McBeath AA. Plantar fascia release for chronic plantar fasciitis in runners. *Am J Sports Med*. 1983;11(4):215-219.

19. Abreu MR, Chung CB, Mendes L, Mohana-Borges A, Trudell D, Resnick D. Plantar calcaneal enthesophytes: new observations regarding sites of origin based on radiographic, MR imaging, anatomic and paleopathologic analysis. *Skeletal Radiol.* 2003;32(1):13-21.
20. Neufeld SK, Cerrato R. Plantar fasciitis: Evaluation and treatment. *J Am Acad Orthop Surg.* 2008;16(6):338-346.
21. Li J, Muehleman C. Anatomic relationship of heel spur to surrounding soft tissues: greater variability than previously reported. *Clin Anat.* 2007;20(8):950-955.
22. Rask MR. Medial plantar neurapraxia (jogger's foot): report of 3 cases. *Clin Orthop Relat Res.* 1978;(134):193-195.
23. Schon LC, Glennon TP, Baxter DE. Heel pain syndrome: electrodiagnostic support for nerve entrapment. *Foot Ankle.* 1993;14(3):129-135.
24. Kerr R, Frey C. MR imaging in tarsal tunnel syndrome. *J Comput Assist Tomogr.* 1991;15(2):280-286.
25. DiGiovanni BF, Nawoczenski DA, Malay DP, et al. Plantar fascia-specific stretching exercise improves outcomes in patients with chronic plantar fasciitis. *J Bone Joint Surg Am.* 2006;88(8):1775-1781.
26. Hofling I, Joukainen A, Venesmaa P, Kroger H. Preliminary experience of a single session of low-energy extracorporeal shock wave treatment for chronic plantar fasciitis. *Foot Ankle Int.* 2008;29(2):150-154.
27. Hyer CF, Vancourt R, Block A. Evaluation of ultrasound-guided extracorporeal shock wave therapy (ESWT) in the treatment of chronic plantar fasciitis. *J Foot Ankle Surg.* 2005;44(2):137-143.
28. Wapner KL, Bordelon RL. Foot and ankle: heel pain. In: DeLee JC, Drez D Jr., Miller MD, eds. *DeLee and Drez's Orthopaedic Sports Medicine: Principles and Practice.* 2nd ed. Philadelphia, PA: W.B. Saunders; 2003:2457-2472.
29. Kantor B, McKenna CJ, Caccitolo JA, et al. Transmyocardial and percutaneous myocardial revascularization: current and future role in the treatment of coronary artery disease. *Mayo Clin Proc.* 1999;74(6):585-592.
30. Ochiai N, Tasto JP, Ohtori S, Takahashi N, Moriya H, Amiel D. Nerve regeneration after radiofrequency application. *Am J Sports Med.* 2007;35(11):1940-1944.
31. Cheung JT, An KN, Zhang M. Consequences of partial and total plantar fascia release: a finite element study. *Foot Ankle Int.* 2006;27(2):125-132.
32. Murphy GA, Pneumaticos SG, Kamaric E, Noble PC, Trevino SG, Baxter DE. Biomechanical consequences of sequential plantar fascia release. *Foot Ankle Int.* 1998;19(3):149-152.

12

Toe Pain and Deformity

Aaron T. Scott, MD

Introduction

Hallux valgus is a common deformity of the great toe that is characterized by lateral deviation of the proximal phalanx at the metatarsophalangeal (MTP) joint, a painfully prominent medial eminence, and a variable degree of pronation of the toe. The common term for this deformity, *bunion*, is derived from the Latin *bunio* which means *turnip*. The etiology is often multifactorial and involves both intrinsic and extrinsic factors. On the lateral side of the foot, a similar deformity can occur with the fifth toe and is commonly referred to as a *bunionette* deformity or a *tailor's bunion*. Treatment of both conditions is

Hurwitz SR, Parekh SG. *Musculoskeletal Examination of the Foot and Ankle: Making the Complex Simple* (pp. 214-232). © 2012 SLACK Incorporated.

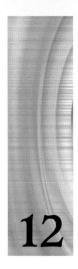

initially nonoperative, with surgery reserved for recalcitrant cases.

Common deformities of the lesser toes include hammer toes, claw toes, mallet toes, and crossover toes. Each of these postural abnormalities may occur in isolation or in association with hallux valgus, and although they may arise as a part of a disease complex or a neuromuscular condition, inappropriate footwear plays a large role in their formation. Deformities of the lesser toes may be flexible or rigid, and this distinction guides surgical management should nonoperative measures fail.

History

A thorough history is essential when evaluating a patient with a bunion deformity, despite the fact that the diagnosis is usually quite apparent. The most common complaint is pain overlying the prominent medial eminence, but other common complaints include pain beneath the medial sesamoid, pain localized to the first MTP joint, cutaneous nerve irritation, difficulty with shoe wear, activity limitations, and cosmetic concerns over the appearance of the foot.[1-3] Associated concerns of lesser toe pain and deformity must also be addressed. Patients with bunionette deformities typically present with complaints of pain overlying the prominent lateral aspect of the fifth metatarsal head, difficulties with shoe wear, and discomfort from thick callus formation.[4-6]

Patients with lesser toe deformities may present with specific complaints such as painful callus formation on the dorsal aspect of the proximal interphalangeal (PIP) joints with hammer toes or claw toes, or pain at the tip of the toe with a mallet toe deformity.[7-9] These complaints are often exacerbated with shoe wear and dissipate when the patient goes barefoot. Other patients may have more vague complaints of forefoot discomfort and have a difficult time localizing the area of pathology (Table 12-1). Pain localized to a lesser MTP joint may be a sign of synovitis,[10,11] a condition that can potentially result in instability of the joint and multiplanar deformity as the surrounding soft tissue restraints become attenuated or may be associated with an osteochondrosis of a lesser metatarsal

Table 12-1

HELPFUL HINTS

Condition	*Description*	*Typical Patient Complaints*
Bunion (hallux valgus)	Valgus alignment of hallux at MTP joint; prominent medial eminence; pronation of great toe	Tenderness over medial eminence; cosmetic concerns over appearance; difficulty with shoewear
Bunionette	Medial deviation of fifth toe at MTP joint; prominent lateral eminence	Tenderness over lateral eminence exacerbated by shoewear; thick callus formation
Hammer toe	PIP flexion; secondary extension at MTP and DIP joints	Painful callus formation over dorsal PIP joint; plantar pain under associated metatarsal head secondary to distal displacement of fat pad
Claw toe	MTP extension; PIP and DIP flexion	Painful callus formation over dorsal PIP joint; plantar pain under associated metatarsal head secondary to distal displacement of fat pad
Mallet toe	DIP flexion	Painful callus on dorsal aspect of DIP joint or at tip of toe
MTP synovitis/ instability	MTP joint inflammation; long-standing disease may lead to capsuloligamentous attenuation and angular deformity at MTP joint	MTP pain and tenderness; deformities such as floating toes or crossover toes
Morton's neuroma	Entrapment neuropathy involving a plantar digital nerve	Vague forefoot or web space pain; subjective sensation of walking on a stone or other foreign object
Freiberg's infraction	Osteochondrosis of a lesser metatarsal head; may see articular collapse on plain radiographs	Vague MTP pain
Intractable plantar keratosis (IPK)	Hyperkeratotic tissue proliferation (callus) on plantar aspect of foot usually under a metatarsal head	Thick, painful plantar callus; easily localized

head, a condition known as a Freiberg's infraction.[11] Burning pain that radiates into a web space and is associated with the abnormal sensation of a foreign object or "knot" on the plantar aspect of the foot may alert the practitioner to the presence of a Morton's neuroma.[12] Finally, many patients present with pain directly plantar to a metatarsal head. This pain is often labeled as the generic *metatarsalgia* and is usually due to fat pad atrophy, distal displacement of the normal fat pad by a hammer toe or claw toe deformity, or an abnormal bony prominence that can subsequently lead to a recalcitrant, painful, thickened callus commonly referred to as an IPK.

Whether the pain and deformity affects the great toe, the lesser toes, or both, certain key elements should be gleaned during the initial history taking. Patients should be questioned regarding the types of shoes they typically wear, any shoe wear modifications that they have tried, and whether their condition is aggravated or relieved with the wearing of shoes. Prior surgeries on the feet should be noted, and a detailed medical history should focus on conditions known to be associated with toe deformities, such as rheumatoid arthritis, osteoarthritis, gout, diabetes, neuromuscular disorders, and lower extremity trauma.[3,5,11] Occupational and recreational demands should be reviewed, and any activity limitations should be recorded. Finally, it is absolutely essential to determine what the patient's expectations are regarding treatment, whether it is nonoperative or operative. This is important because a patient may have the unrealistic belief that he or she will have no activity or shoe wear limitations following treatment.

Examination

Patients with pain and deformity of the hallux and lesser toes are examined in both the standing and seated positions. Limb alignment and overall posture of the foot are evaluated, and abnormalities are carefully noted. A thorough neurovascular exam focusing on pulses, capillary refill, sensation, and motor function is critically important as deviations from the norm may influence the selection of treatment options or the outcome following a particular treatment modality.

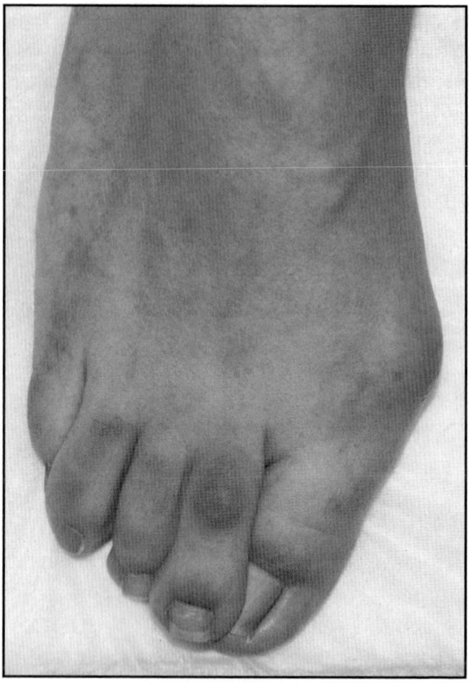

Figure 12-1. Clinical appearance of a bunion deformity with associated second toe overlap.

Examination of bunions and bunionette deformities begins with standing inspection. The degree of deformity and the presence of calluses are noted, as are any associated central lesser toe deformities (Figure 12-1). Palpation may elicit tenderness over the medial eminence, sesamoids, dorsal first MTP joint, or along the dorsal or plantar cutaneous nerves of the hallux. Similarly, patients with bunionette deformities may exhibit tenderness overlying the lateral eminence secondary to callus formation or bursal inflammation. Range of motion (ROM) of the first MTP and first metatarsocuneiform joints is determined and is compared to the contralateral side. Decreased ROM and pain during ROM of the first MTP joint may be a sign of hallux rigidus, but the significance of first metatarsocuneiform hypermobility remains controversial.

Lesser toe complaints require a meticulous evaluation as the correct diagnosis can often be ascertained by physical examination methods alone. Hammer toes, claw toes, crossover toes, and mallet toes are determined to be either fixed

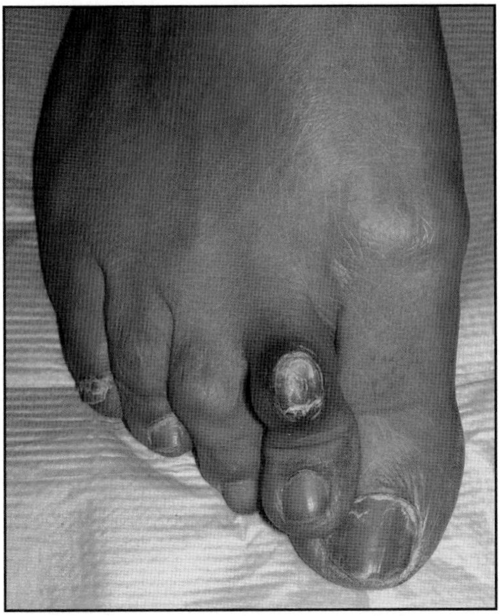

Figure 12-2. Painful dorsal PIP joint callus secondary to a hammer toe deformity.

or flexible, a distinction that guides surgical management should nonoperative measures fail.[7,11,13] Calluses may be present dorsally over the PIP (Figure 12-2) or at the toe tips. The lesser MTP joints are evaluated for tenderness and instability, both of which may be indicative of a synovitis. This instability is best determined by performing a toe Lachman's test[7,11] in which the examiner grasps the metatarsal neck between the index finger and thumb with one hand while grasping the proximal phalanx with the opposite index finger and thumb, and attempts to effect a dorsal subluxation of the joint (Table 12-2). Tenderness between metatarsal heads is often associated with a Morton's neuroma, and if difficulty distinguishing between MTP synovitis and a Morton's neuroma arises, one may attempt a diagnostic injection into the affected web space (see Table 12-2). Patients with metatarsalgia display tenderness on the plantar aspect of their metatarsal heads secondary to fat pad atrophy or distal displacement of the fat pad commonly seen with claw toes, or secondary to a bony prominence that may result in an IPK (callus).

Table 12-2

METHODS FOR EXAMINATION

Confusing Diagnosis	*Distinguishing Exam Techniques*
MTP synovitis/ instability versus Morton's neuroma	1. Toe Lachman's: Examiner grasps proximal phalanx of involved toe with one hand while grasping metatarsal with other hand. The ability to dorsally sublux the MTP joint is associated with instability (and synovitis) (Figure 12-3A). 2. Mulder's click: Examiner applies dorsal pressure to the involved plantar web space while simultaneously compressing all 5 metatarsal heads together. An audible "click" and reproduction of the patients pain are felt to be diagnostic of a Morton's (interdigital) neuroma (Figure 12-3B). 3. Diagnostic injection: Examiner injects 1 mL of 1% lidocaine solution into the affected web space from dorsal to plantar between metatarsal necks. A 25-gauge needle should be used and the anesthetic should be injected just deep to the plantar skin as the nerve lies in a relatively plantar location. Pain relief suggests the possibility of a Morton's neuroma. Alternatively the injection can be placed into a lesser MTP joint (Figure 12-3C).
IPK versus Plantar wart	1. Paring: Shaving of a plantar wart with a #15 blade will reveal punctate bleeding, whereas shaving of an IPK will not. 2. Pinch test: Plantar warts are most tender when pinched between the thumb and index finger, whereas IPKs are most tender when a direct pressure is applied from plantar to dorsal.

PATHOANATOMY

It is generally accepted that the formation of a bunion deformity occurs as a result of both extrinsic and intrinsic factors.[1-3] The primary extrinsic factor is felt to be constrictive shoe wear,[14] whereas commonly cited intrinsic factors include

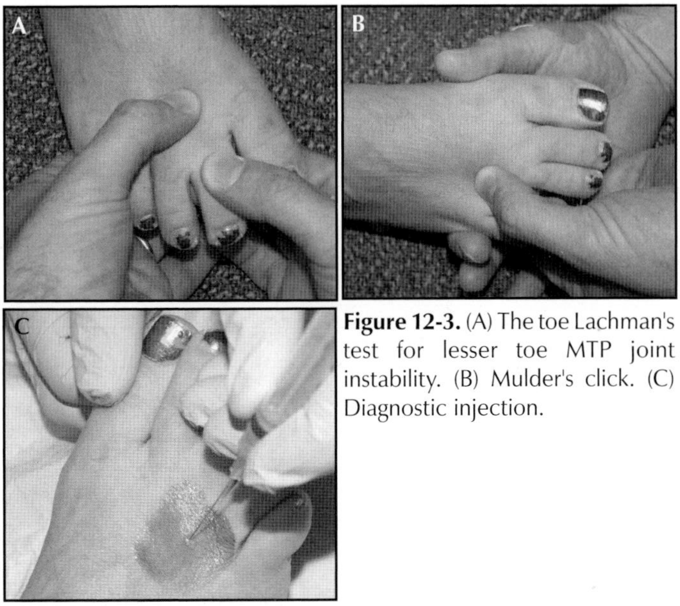

Figure 12-3. (A) The toe Lachman's test for lesser toe MTP joint instability. (B) Mulder's click. (C) Diagnostic injection.

a family history of bunions, flatfoot deformity, a round first metatarsal head, and possibly, hypermobility of the first metatarsocuneiform joint.[1,2] Regardless of the precise interplay between these intrinsic and extrinsic elements, it is the valgus force at the first MTP joint that sets in motion this complex and progressive deformity.[2,3] As the proximal phalanx drifts into a valgus position, the first metatarsal head is pushed medially, thus creating a varus malalignment of the first metatarsal shaft. As the magnitude of the deformity increases, the medial capsule becomes attenuated while lateral capsular structures become contracted, and the adductor hallucis is placed at a biomechanical advantage, thus further perpetuating the deformity. Additional findings include pronation of the hallux secondary to overpull of the adductor hallucis (Figure 12-4) and medial displacement of the first metatarsal head from its normal position overlying the sesamoid complex. Similar to its medial counterpart, the development of a bunionette deformity is felt to be multifactorial with the extrinsic culprit being an increased angle between the fourth and fifth metatarsal shafts.[4,5]

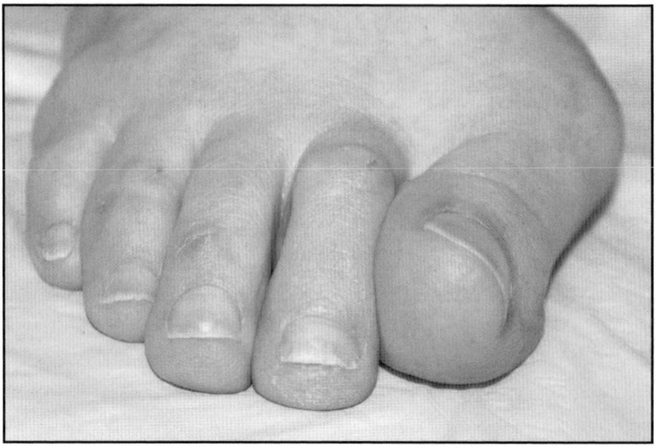

Figure 12-4. Pronation of the hallux secondary to overpull of the adductor hallucis. Note the internally rotated nail of the great toe in comparison to the nails of the lesser toes.

Lesser MTP joint instability is most common in the second toe[7] and is rarely the result of a single traumatic event. The typical scenario is that repetitive overload of the joint results in synovitis with eventual attenuation of the capsuloligamentous restraints.[11,15] This repetitive overload is commonly the result of a hallux valgus deformity with its increased load transfer to the second ray, but may also be associated with a short first metatarsal, long second metatarsal, or high-heeled shoes with a narrow toe box as some authors have suggested.[15] As the plantar plate becomes attenuated, sagittal plane instability is lost, and subluxation or dislocation may ensue (Figure 12-5). When attenuation of the collateral ligaments occurs in combination with weakening of the plantar plate, the common "crossover" deformity that is seen in association with bunions may develop.[9,11,15,16]

By definition, a mallet toe demonstrates a flexion contracture of the distal interphalangeal (DIP) joint with relatively normal PIP and MTP joints, whereas hammer toes display a flexion contracture of the PIP joint, often with secondary

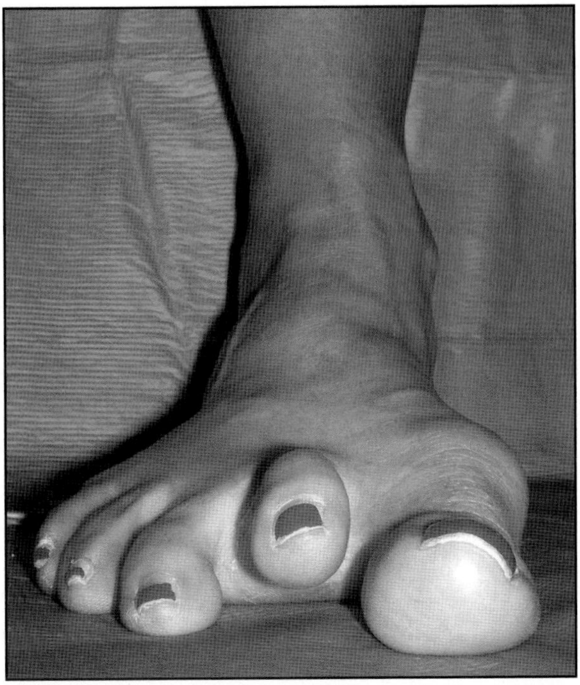

Figure 12-5. Long-standing synovitis may lead to attenuation of the plantar plate with resulting sagittal plane instability and a "floating toe."

extension at the DIP and MTP joints.[7] Mallet toes and hammer toes are both felt to occur most often secondary to shoes with constrictive toe boxes.[17] Each of these deformities is seen more often in the longest toe and represents the position that the toe must assume to fit within the confines of the shoe. Over time, a contracture may develop and the initially flexible deformity can potentially become rigid, or "fixed." These deformities can also be seen in association with a neuromuscular disorder, and classically involves multiple toes on both feet. By definition, a claw toe involves a hyperextension at the MTP joint with secondary flexion contractures at the PIP and DIP joints caused by a muscular imbalance between the intrinsic and extrinsic muscles of the lower leg and foot.[17] The normal function of the intrinsic muscles of the foot (the interossei and lumbricals) is to provide flexion at the MTP joint while simultaneously extending the PIP and DIP joints. However, when these intrinsic muscles become weak, as is often the case in certain neuromuscular conditions, they may become overpowered by the extrinsic extensor tendons at the MTP joint and by the flexor tendons at the PIP and DIP joints, thereby leading to the abnormal posture of the claw toe. As the MTP hyperextension deformity of a hammer toe or claw toe progresses, the normal plantar fat pad migrates distally, thus uncovering the plantar aspect of the corresponding metatarsal head, an occurrence that may lead to metatarsalgia and callus formation.[7]

Imaging

Plain radiographs are essential in the work-up of any patients with toe pain and deformity. The patient should be full weight bearing for these films and the standard 3 views (anteroposterior [AP], lateral, and oblique) will usually suffice in most instances. The examination of radiographs taken for the painful bunion begins with evaluation of the MTP joint for degenerative arthritis or incongruity and an assessment of sesamoid position.[2,18] The evaluation then progresses to the measurement of several key angles.[18] Among these are the angle formed by the longitudinal axes of the first metatarsal and proximal phalanx (hallux valgus (HV) angle in Figure 12-6), angle formed by the longitudinal axes of the first and second metatarsal shafts (1-2 intermetatarsal [IM] angle in Figure 12-7), the angle between the longitudinal axes of the proximal and distal phalanges (hallux interphalangeal angle in Figure 12-8), and the lateral deviation of the distal first metatarsal articular surface from the axis of the first metatarsal shaft (distal metatarsal articular angle [DMAA] in Figure 12-9).

Bunionette deformities have been classified into 3 types based on radiographic criteria that include the measurement

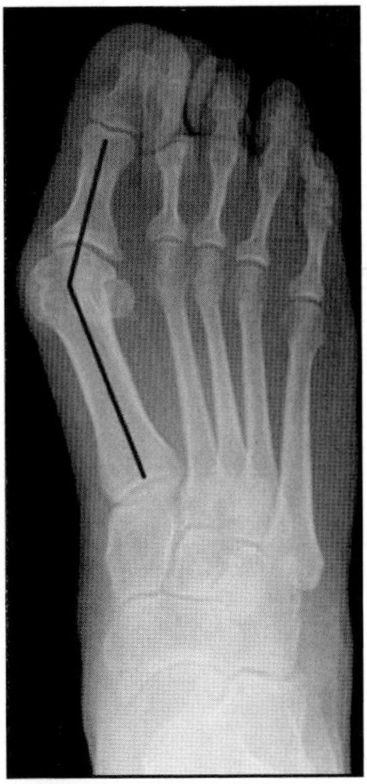

Figure 12-6. Hallux valgus angle.

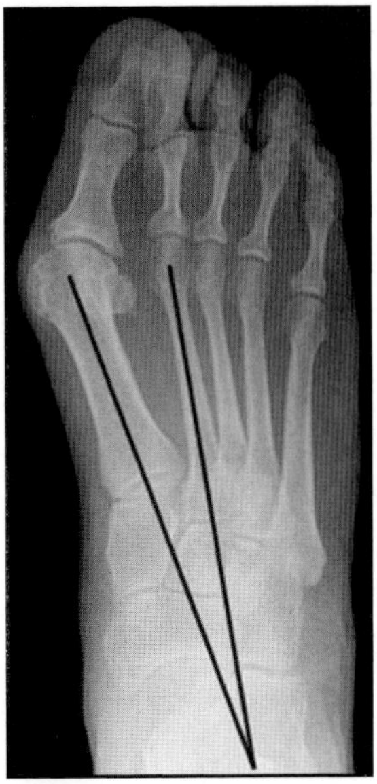

Figure 12-7. 1-2 IM angle.

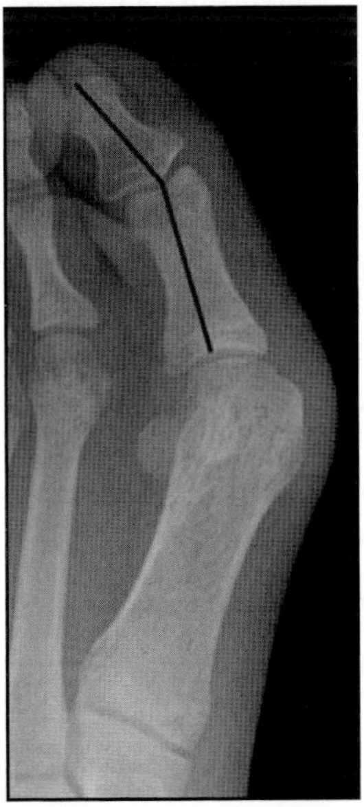

Figure 12-8. Hallux interphalangeal angle.

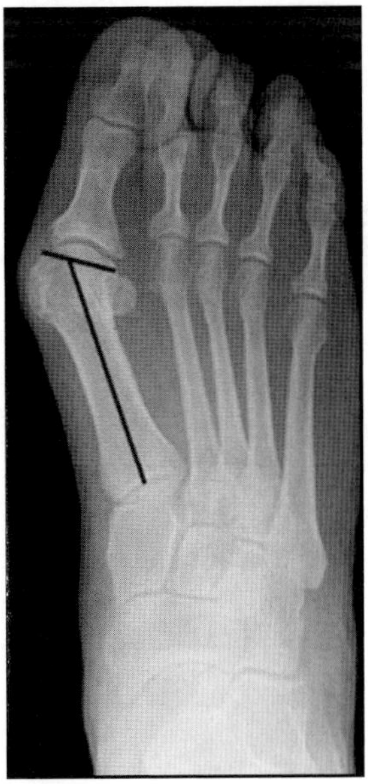

Figure 12-9. DMAA.

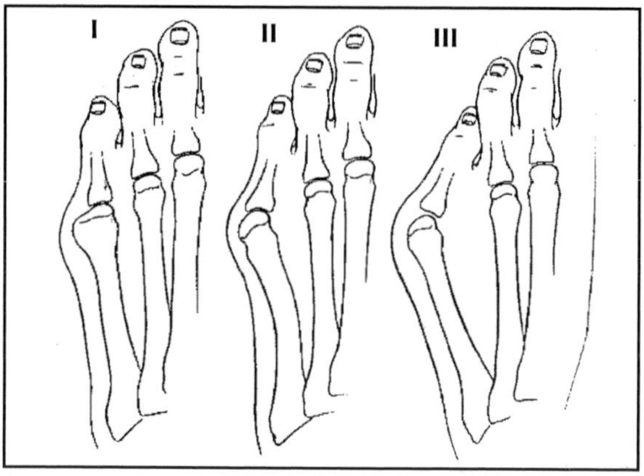

Figure 12-10. Bunionette classification. (This figure was published in *Foot and Ankle Disorders*, Vol. 1, Myerson, MS, Disorders and deformities of the lesser toes, p. 336, Copyright Saunders Elsevier [2000].)

of 2 angles[4] (Figure 12-10). The first of these angles is the MTP-5 angle (Figure 12-11), which is the angle formed by the longitudinal axes of the fifth metatarsal and proximal phalanx (average 10.2 degrees in the normal foot). The second important angle is the 4-5 IM angle (Figure 12-12), which averages 6.2 degrees in the normal foot and is determined by measuring the angle between the longitudinal axes of the fourth and fifth metatarsal shafts. Type I bunionette deformities possess an enlarged lateral eminence with normal MTP-5 and 4-5 IM angles. Type II deformities possess an abnormal lateral bowing of the fifth metatarsal shaft with an associated increase in the MTP-5 angle. Finally, Type III bunionette deformities are characterized by an increased 4-5 IM angle.

When evaluating radiographs obtained for the work-up of a lesser toe deformity, one must not overlook abnormalities of the hallux, midfoot, and hindfoot as these may contribute to problems arising in the lesser toes. Despite the fact that hammer toes, claw toes, and mallet toes may be readily apparent on lateral radiographs, careful attention must be paid to the AP and oblique x-rays. When assessing the AP view, it is especially important to note any length discrepancies between metatarsals and any incongruency present at any of the MTP joints

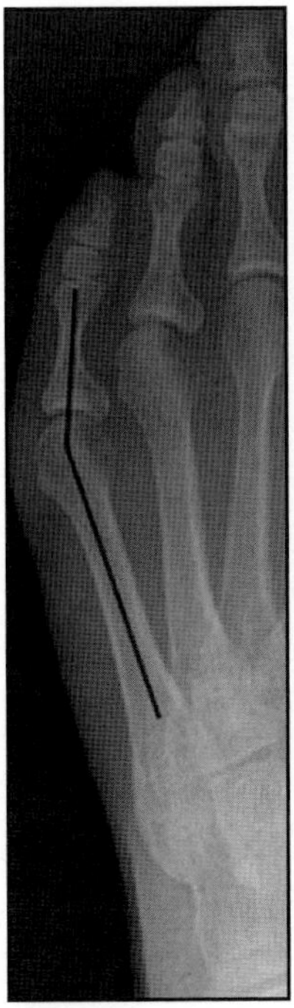

Figure 12-11. MTP-5 angle.

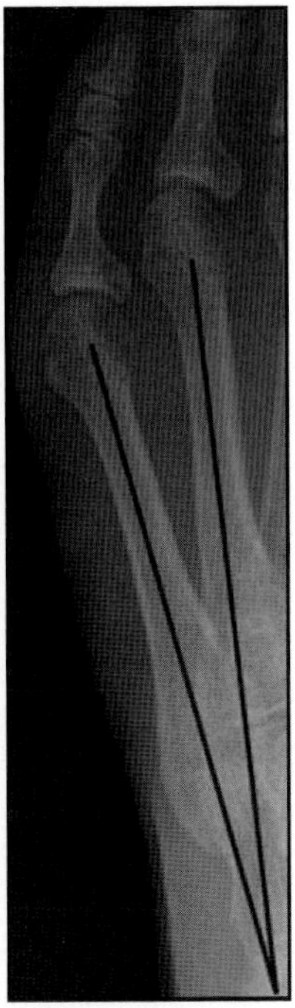

Figure 12-12. 4-5 IM angle.

(Figure 12-13). The oblique views are especially helpful when combined with the AP view for evaluating lesser metatarsal heads for subchondral collapse seen in Freiberg's infraction or in assessing a metatarsal for stress fracture.

Treatment

The management of the symptomatic bunion deformity begins with nonsurgical modalities,[19] the most important of which is shoe wear modifications.[2] Patients should be encouraged to wear shoes with a wider toe box or open-toe shoes to reduce pressure over a tender medial eminence, and patients with associated sesamoid pain may benefit from custom orthotics with a depression under this region. Other nonsurgical appliances such as bunion splints and toe spacers

Figure 12-13. Lesser toe MTP synovitis may lead to instability, subluxation, and even dislocation. Note the frank dislocation of the second MTP joint.

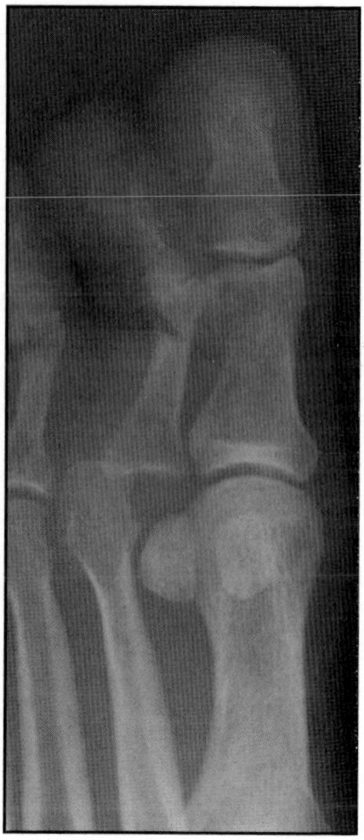

have very little long-term utility in the nonoperative treatment of this condition and have not been shown to reverse the deformity.[2] The surgeon treating a patient who has failed nonoperative management has over 130 surgical procedures at his or her disposal.[20] Although this is a daunting number and a thorough discussion of the surgical management is beyond the scope of this text, certain surgical principles guide the selection of the appropriate procedure[18] and many of these operations have identical indications. In general, mild deformities (HV angle <30 degrees and 1-2 IM angle <13 degrees) with an incongruent MTP joint are managed with a distal first metatarsal osteotomy such as a distal chevron procedure with resection of the medial eminence and an imbrication of the medial joint capsule.[18,21] Moderate (HV angle 30 to 40 degrees and 1-2 IM angle 13 to 20 degrees) and severe (HV angle >40 degrees and 1-2 IM angle >20 degrees) deformities are typically treated with one of numerous proximal first metatarsal osteotomies and release of the contracted lateral soft tissues of the first MTP joint along with a medial eminence resection.[18,21] Another option for the severe bunion or the arthritic bunion is a first MTP arthrodesis[18] (fusion). Finally, patients with congruent MTP joints (increased DMAA) will require some form of closing wedge osteotomy of the distal first metatarsal to reduce the lateral angulation of the articular surface.[21]

Conversion to shoes with a wider toe box remains the cornerstone of the conservative management of the symptomatic bunionette deformity, but custom orthotics designed to relieve pressure under the fifth metatarsal head and shaving of the thickened calluses may prove to be helpful adjuncts.[5] Patients failing nonsurgical management may benefit from surgical intervention guided by the previously presented classification scheme. Because angular measurements are normal in patients with Type I deformities, surgery entails resection of the prominent lateral eminence with imbrication of the lateral fifth MTP capsule.[4] Type II and III bunionette deformities require an osteotomy through the distal or midshaft fifth metatarsal in addition to the lateral eminence resection to gain adequate correction.[4,6]

Although conservative management of hammer toes, claw toes, and mallet toes will not permanently correct the deformity, substantial symptomatic relief can be attained without surgery[10,11] (Figure 12-14). The pain secondary to dorsal pressure over a lesser PIP joint of a hammer toe or claw toe can often be relieved with extra-depth shoes or silicone toe sleeves, and toe crests allow the painful tip of a mallet toe to be elevated off the ground. Other nonoperative options include taping or toe slings to realign the flexible hammer toe or claw toe and metatarsal pads or metatarsal bars positioned proximal to a metatarsal head to relieve pressure and the metatarsalgia. Surgical treatment for recalcitrant cases is guided by the relative flexibility of the deformity. Flexible hammer toes and claw toes are commonly treated by transferring the flexor digitorum longus tendon to the dorsal aspect of the proximal phalanx, thereby reducing the flexion deformity at the PIP joint while simultaneously bringing the MTP joint out of hyperextension.[7] The flexible mallet toe requires little more than a percutaneous release of the flexor digitorum longus tendon.[10] Fixed hammer toes and claw toes will not respond to isolated tendon

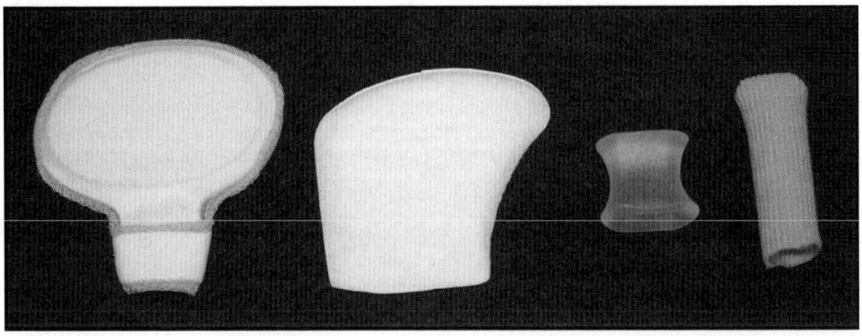

Figure 12-14. Appliances commonly used in the nonoperative management of lesser toe pain and deformity. From left to right: hammer toe sling, metatarsal pad, toe spacer, and silicone sleeve.

transfers and will require both soft tissue and bony procedures. For the fixed hammer toe deformity, surgery generally entails an extensor tendon lengthening and dorsal capsulotomy to release the extension contracture of the MTP joint in combination with a PIP arthrodesis or proximal phalangeal head resection to treat the fixed flexion deformity of the PIP joint.[13,17,22] Surgical treatment of the rigid claw toe deformity parallels that of the rigid hammer toe, unless a severe contracture, subluxation, or dislocation of the MTP joint exists, which will necessitate a metatarsal shortening osteotomy to decompress the joint.[10,17] The fixed mallet toe will require a DIP arthrodesis or resection of the middle phalangeal condyles.[10]

Although taping and toe slings may provide the patient with some symptomatic relief of the pain associated with an MTP synovitis, instability, or crossover deformity, nonoperative treatment rarely provides a permanent solution.[7,10] Surgical treatment for MTP synovitis or instability is guided by the relative severity of the condition. Despite the fact that a recalcitrant case of MTP synovitis can be treated with MTP joint capsulotomy and débridement,[11] most patients present with deformity and instability requiring a more extensive procedure. Mild or moderate cases of instability can often be treated with extensor tendon Z-lengthening, dorsal capsulotomy, MTP joint débridement, release of the contracted collateral ligament, and tightening of the attenuated collateral ligament.[7,10] A flexor-to-extensor tendon transfer as described for the flexible hammer toe or claw toe may also be added to act as a checkrein to dorsal subluxation.[23,24] However, severe subluxation, dislocation, or a crossover toe deformity may require the addition of a metatarsal shortening osteotomy or an extensor tendon transfer to control angular deformity.[17,23,25]

Conclusion

Pain and deformity involving the hallux and lesser toes are not rare. They may occur in isolation or as a component of a broader medical condition, and the impact of improper shoe wear cannot be overemphasized. Initial treatment generally involves nonsurgical interventions such as shoe wear modifications, orthotics, or the use of other appliances that may provide some symptomatic relief, but rarely effect a cure. Surgery may be indicated for recalcitrant cases and is highly dependent upon the magnitude or rigidity of the deformity as determined by the physical examination and critical evaluation of the plain radiographs.

References

1. Coughlin MJ, Jones CP. Hallux valgus: demographics, etiology, and radiographic assessment. *Foot Ankle Int*. 2007;28(7):759-777.
2. Easley ME, Trnka H-J. Current concepts review: hallux valgus part I: Pathomechanics, clinical assessment, and nonoperative management. *Foot Ankle Int*. 2007;28(5):654-659.
3. Robinson AH, Limbers JP. Modern concepts in the treatment of hallux valgus. *J Bone Joint Surg Br*. 2005;87(8):1038-1045.
4. Cohen BE, Nicholson CW. Bunionette deformity. *J Am Acad Orthop Surg*. 2007;15(5):300-307.
5. Koti M, Maffulli N. Bunionette. *J Bone Joint Surg Am*. 2001;83-A(7):1076-1082.
6. Vienne P, Oesselmann M, Espinosa N, Aschwanden R, Zingg P. Modified Coughlin procedure for surgical treatment of symptomatic tailor's bunion: A prospective followup study of 33 consecutive operations. *Foot Ankle Int*. 2006;27(8):573-580.
7. Coughlin MJ. Common causes of pain in the forefoot in adults. *J Bone Joint Surg Br*. 2000;82(6):781-790.
8. Lancaster SC, Sizensky JA, Young CC. Acute mallet toe. *Clin J Sport Med*. 2008;18(3):298-299.
9. Myerson MS, Shereff MJ. The pathological anatomy of claw and hammer toes. *J Bone Joint Surg Am*. 1989;71(1):45-49.

10. Easley ME, Aydogan U. Lesser toe deformities and bunionettes. In Thordarson DB, ed. *Orthopaedic Surgery Essentials: Foot and Ankle.* Philadelphia, PA: Lippincott Williams and Wilkins; 2004:131-152.
11. Mizel MS, Yodlowski ML. Disorders of the lesser metatarsophalangeal joints. *J Am Acad Orthop Surg.* 1995;3(3):166-173.
12. Morris MA. Morton's metatarsalgia. *Clin Orthop Relat Res.* 1977;(127):203-207.
13. Coughlin MJ, Dorris J, Polk E. Operative repair of the fixed hammertoe deformity. *Foot Ankle Int.* 2000;21(2):94-104.
14. Sim-Fook L, Hodgson AR. A comparison of foot forms among the non-shoe and shoe-wearing Chinese population. *J Bone Joint Surg Am.* 1958;40-A(5):1058-1062.
15. Kaz AJ, Coughlin MJ. Crossover second toe: demographics, etiology, and radiographic assessment. *Foot Ankle Int.* 2007;28(12):1223-1237.
16. Bhatia D, Myerson MS, Curtis MJ, Cunningham BW, Jinnah RH. Anatomical restraints to dislocation of the second metatarsophalangeal joint and assessment of a repair technique. *J Bone Joint Surg Am.* 1994;76(9):1371-1375.
17. Coughlin MJ. Lesser toe deformities. In Coughlin MJ, Mann RA, Saltzman CL, eds. *Surgery of the Foot and Ankle.* Philadelphia, PA: Mosby Incorporated; 2007:363-464.
18. Mann RA. Disorders of the first metatarsophalangeal joint. *J Am Acad Orthop Surg.* 1995;3(1):34-43.
19. Torkki M, Malmivaara A, Seitsalo S, Hoikka V, Laippala P, Paavolainen P. Surgery vs orthosis vs watchful waiting for hallux valgus: a randomized controlled trial. *JAMA.* 2001;285(19):2474-2480.
20. Helal B, Gupta SK, Gojaseni P. Surgery for adolescent hallux valgus. *Acta Orthop Scand.* 1974;45(2):271-295.
21. Easley ME, Trnka H-J. Current concepts review: Hallux valgus part II: operative treatment. *Foot Ankle Int.* 2007;28(6):748-758.
22. O'Kane C, Kilmartin T. Review of proximal interphalangeal joint excision arthroplasty for the correction of second hammer toe deformity in 100 cases. *Foot Ankle Int.* 2005;26(4):320-325.
23. Haddad SL, Sabbagh RC, Resch S, Myerson B, Myerson MS. Results of flexor-to-extensor and extensor brevis tendon transfer for correction of the crossover second toe deformity. *Foot Ankle Int.* 1999;20(12):781-788.
24. Myerson MS, Jung H-G. The role of toe flexor-to-extensor transfer in correcting metatarsophalangeal joint instability of the second toe. *Foot Ankle Int.* 2005;26:675-679.
25. Trnka H-J, Muhlbauer M, Zettl R, Myerson MS, Ritschl P. Comparison of the results of the Weil and Helal osteotomies for the treatment of metatarsalgia secondary to dislocation of the lesser metatarsophalangeal joints. *Foot Ankle Int.* 1999;20(2):72-79.

Financial Disclosures

Dr. Ian Alexander has not disclosed any relevant financial relationships.

Dr. Judith F. Baumhauer is a paid consultant for DJ Orthopaedics, Carticept, Extremity Medical and Biomimetic Therapeutics; receives research support from DJO; is on the Foot and Ankle International Techniques in Foot and Ankle Surgery board; and is a board member for American Orthopaedic Foot and Ankle Society, Orthopaedic Research and Education Foundation, Orthopaedic Education Foundation, Eastern Orthopaedic Association, American Board of Orthopaedic Surgery, and American Board Medical Specialties.

Dr. Wayne Berberian has not disclosed any relevant financial relationships.

Dr. Eric Breitbart has no financial or proprietary interest in the materials presented herein.

Dr. Christopher P. Chiodo has no financial or proprietary interest in the materials presented herein.

Dr. Premjit S. Deol has no financial or proprietary interest in the materials presented herein.

Dr. Antonio Gomez-Tristan has no financial or proprietary interest in the materials presented herein.

Dr. Adam T. Groth has no financial or proprietary interest in the materials presented herein.

Dr. Shepard R. Hurwitz has no financial or proprietary interest in the materials presented herein.

Dr. Sheldon Lin is a member of the Scientific Advisory Board of Biomimetics Therapeutics Inc. and TissueGene.

Dr. James Meeker has no financial or proprietary interest in the materials presented herein.

Dr. Samir Mehta has no financial or proprietary interest in the materials presented herein.

Dr. Selene G. Parekh receives a grant from Orthohelix and is a consultant for Biomet, Sonoma Orthopaedics, Kyphon, Memometal, Invuity, and Extremity Medical.

Dr. David I. Pedowitz has not disclosed any relevant financial relationships.

Dr. Terrence M. Philbin has no financial or proprietary interest in the materials presented herein.

Dr. Seth R. Queler has no financial or proprietary interest in the materials presented herein.

Dr. Sudheer Reddy is a consultant for Integra Life Sciences.

Dr. Lew Schon is a consultant for and has an inventor relationship with Tornier.

Dr. Aaron T. Scott has no financial or proprietary interest in the materials presented herein.

Dr. Joshua N. Tennant has no financial or proprietary interest in the materials presented herein.

Dr. Keith Wapner is a consultant for Wright Medical, MMI/Stryker, and Small Bone Innovations and receives institutional support from Hangar, Inc.

Index

ttention Industry Partners!

hether you are interested in buying multiple copies of a book, chapter reprints, looking for something new and different — we are able to accommodate our needs.

ULTIPLE COPIES

attractive discounts starting for purchases as low as 25 copies for single title, SLACK Incorporated will be able to meet all your of your needs.

HAPTER REPRINTS

ACK Incorporated is able to offer the chapters you want in a format that ll lead to success. Bound with an attractive cover, use the chapters that e a fit specifically for your company. Available for quantities of 100 or more.

USTOMIZE

ACK Incorporated is able to create a specialized custom version of any our products specifically for your company.

ase contact the Marketing Communications Director for further details on multiple py purchases, chapter reprints, or custom printing at 1-800-257-8290 or 1-856-848-1000.

ease note all conditions are subject to change.

SLACK®
NCORPORATED
Health Care Books and Journals • 6900 Grove Road • Thorofare, NJ 08086

1-800-257-8290
ax: 1-856-848-6091
-mail: **orders@slackinc.com**
ODE: 328

www.slackbooks.com